Physics in Medical Ultrasound

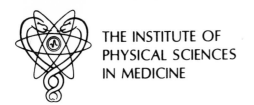

THE INSTITUTE OF
PHYSICAL SCIENCES
IN MEDICINE

Physics in Medical Ultrasound

Edited by J A Evans

Report No. 47

© The Institute of Physical Sciences in Medicine 1986
47 Belgrave Square
London SW1X 8QX

ISBN 0 904181 42 1

Published by the Institute of Physical Sciences in Medicine,
47 Belgrave Square, London SW1X 8QX, England

In September 1982, the Hospital Physicists' Association (HPA) formed the Institute of Physical Sciences in Medicine (IPSM) as a Company limited by guarantee. The Institute, which was granted Charitable Status in April 1984, was established to promote for public benefit the advancement of physics and allied physical sciences applied to medicine and biology, and to advance public education in this field. For these purposes it has been decided, among other things, to transfer the publications activities of the Association to the Institute as from 1st January, 1985. In future, therefore, all books and booklets will be published by the Institute of Physical Sciences in Medicine.

Printed by Bocardo Press Limited, Oxford

CONTENTS

PREFACE

Few techniques can have changed as rapidly as medical ultrasound during the last twenty years. The images obtained from scanners even five years ago look poor in comparison with those of today. This change in technology has brought with it significant changes in the nature and numbers of the personnel involved. Gone are the days when it was impossible to run a hospital ultrasound service without a physicist standing by to adjust the knobs, help interpret the images and repair the machine after one of its frequent breakdowns. Ultrasound scanners are now to be found in most district hospitals and the service is often provided without any direct Medical Physics involvement.

These changes have forced physicists working in ultrasound to re-examine their role. Since Medical Physicists as a group traditionally have tried to stay on the growing edge of subjects, the increased routine use of ultrasound by medical and para-medical groups should be seen as an opportunity rather than a threat. That this opportunity has been seized is amply demonstrated in this booklet.

The scientific challenges laid down by medical ultrasonics remain as great as ever. Fundamental understanding of the interaction of ultrasound with biological materials is still lacking and hence the image forming process cannot be described as fully understood. Therefore quality control is a subject receiving considerable attention. The recent controversy over ultrasound safety has provided an added stimulus for studies on biological effects and output measurements. These topics are well represented here.

On a more clinical note, Doppler ultrasound seems finally to have come of age, alongside its imaging siblings. However, in this case the interpretation of the output remains very much in the province of the clinical physicist. Whether this will remain so is a matter for crystal ball gazing but it is clear that many interesting questions remain.

This booklet represents the proceedings of a meeting held at the Hatfield College, University of Durham, on July 11–12, 1985. It was organised by the Ultrasound Topic Group of the IPSM, and was co-sponsored by the British Medical Ultrasound Society, the Physical Acoustics Group of the Institute of Physics, and the Institute of Acoustics. It is hoped that the range of topics covered includes most aspects of the 'state-of-the-art' in medical ultrasound physics in 1985. If it provides a stimulus to delve further with enthusiasm then it will have fulfilled its purpose.

The task of organising the meeting fell mainly to Dr Kevin Martin, the Local Organiser, and he is to be commended for his tremendous efforts. I would also like to record my thanks to the other members of the Topic Group who all made a significant contribution; Mr Geoff Cusick, Dr David Evans and Mr David McHugh. Awards of thanks are also due to all the authors who provided their copy so promptly and made the editorial task much easier, and to Mr Robert Price for his help with proof reading.

Finally, it is worth pointing out that the views expressed in the papers are those of the individual authors. In any lively 'state-of-the-art' meeting there will be controversy. It is left to the reader to decide which views to accept and which to challenge.

J A Evans
Leeds 1986

A Review of Recent Experimental Evidence on the Effects of Diagnostic Ultrasound on Tissue

Mary Dyson
Department of Anatomy, United Medical and Dental Schools of Guy's and St Thomas's Hospitals, Guy's Hospital, London SE1 9RT

1.1 Introduction

Ultrasound is of great value as a diagnostic agent and, as currently applied, has an excellent safety record. Confidence in the efficacy and safety of diagnostic ultrasound is such that in many hospitals consideration is being given to its routine use during pregnancy. However, the use of any interrogative agent can never be free from risk, for such agents affect the object interrogated; this is inevitable if information is to be obtained. What matters is whether diagnostic ultrasound affects in a significant manner the patients it is used to examine. Provided that the risk of this is small in comparison to the benefit derived by the patient from the use of diagnostic ultrasound, then it is in the patient's best interests that the investigation be carried out, since it may be far more hazardous for it not to be. Assessment of the degree of risk involved has to be made, and this can only be achieved satisfactorily if the manner in which ultrasound affects the cells and tissues of the body is understood.

Ultrasound can produce a wide variety of effects on the structure and function of cells and tissues[1,2]. Although many of these effects have been induced by ultrasound at intensity levels above those used diagnostically, the thresholds for them have generally not been determined, and it is possible that some may also occur following the use of diagnostic ultrasound in certain circumstances. Since the possibility of such risk cannot be ignored, in the interests of safety a hypothetical risk should be presumed, and steps taken to reduce this as much as possible. In particular, evidence of changes in cells and tissues following exposure

Table 1.1 Intensity levels currently used in medical ultrasound.

Category	Approximate intensity range (SATA)* in mW cm^{-2}
Surgical	10,000
Therapeutic	3,000–100
Diagnostic	
Perivascular Doppler	500– 50
Other varieties**	50– 0.1

(Modified from Table 5.1 in NCRP Report 74)

* SATA = spatial average, temporal average.
** For pulse-echo devices the duty factor is such that the spatial average, temporal peak intensity (SATP) is typically 1,000 times the SATA intensity.

to diagnostic ultrasound should be examined critically, the significance of these changes in relationship to the continued safe use of ultrasound assessed and, where appropriate, methods of avoiding them established.

Although currently used diagnostic levels of ultrasound (*table 1.1*) are not generally considered to produce clinically significant effects, the levels used therapeutically and surgically affect cell behaviour in a clinically significant manner[3]. Many of the cellular effects recorded following the use of relatively low levels of ultrasound therapy (for example, 100 mW cm^{-2}, spatial average, temporal average, at 3 MHz), are nonthermal in origin[4], and appear to involve changes in the permeability of the cell membrane. They include alteration of cell motility and the stimulation of protein synthesis and secretion, — changes which could affect the progress of embryogenesis. Although the output of some diagnostic instruments may overlap with that of some therapeutic devices, attenuation by the maternal tissues ensures a considerable reduction in the intensity of ultrasound to which an embryo or fetus may be exposed, when compared with the output from the transducer[5]. Even so, particular caution is advisable if such machines are used early in pregnancy, when exposure of the uterus should be minimised. The levels used surgically, where the intention is to produce localised tissue destruction, are too much in excess of those used in diagnosis to be of relevance in any consideration of the safe use of diagnostic ultrasound.

1.2   Evidence for adverse effects

Recent evidence of ultrasonically-induced effects which have a bearing on the continued safe use of diagnostic ultrasound can be grouped according to its source:

1.   Human (epidemiological studies)
2.   Experimental animals (*in vivo* studies)
3.   Mammalian cells (*in vitro* studies)

1.2.1   Human epidemiology

Although practising physicians have not identified any adverse effects arising directly from the diagnostic use of ultrasound, the fact that it can produce effects on animals *in vivo* and on mammalian cells *in vitro* under certain circumstances (see below) has caused safety to remain a matter of considerable concern, particularly for exposures involving the embryo or fetus. Epidemiological investigations have proved difficult in the past, mainly because of the problem of matching exposed and unexposed groups of patients, since those examined with diagnostic ultrasound generally differed in health from those who were not.

A national survey of clinical users carried out by the Environmental Health Directorate of Canada[6], published in 1980, revealed that out of 1,200,000 examinations during 1977, involving 340,000 patients, only one adverse effect was reported, and that unspecified in nature. Although the results of such large surveys are reassuring, it should be appreciated that even surveys of this size are not well suited to the detection of small changes in the rate of occurrence of the more common abnormalities, and that subtle effects such as minor behavioural changes and long-term delayed effects can escape detection.

2

The positive finding by Moore *et al* in 1982[7] of a decrease in mean birth weight in babies exposed to diagnostic ultrasound prenatally has caused considerable interest. Analysis of the accumulated records from 1968 to 1972 of 2,135 single births, half of which were of children exposed to ultrasound, revealed an association between low birth weight and ultrasound. However, the data were analysed several years after collection, and the records available were not sufficiently detailed to allow adjustments to be made for the physical size of the parents, nor for the health of the mother, nor for whether the mother smoked — all factors which could affect birth weight.

In 1983 Stark *et al*[8], using a subset of cases from the same data base as that used in the previous study by Moore *et al*, analysed the records of children exposed prenatally to ultrasound and of 381 matched controls. In addition to birth weight, 16 other variables were compared, including Apgar scores, congenital abnormalities, hearing, visual acuity, colour vision and behaviour. No significant differences were found between the exposed and unexposed children. These results cast doubt upon the clinical significance of those presented earlier by Moore *et al*[7].

Continuous Doppler ultrasound monitoring may be used for many hours during labour, and any report of an increase in erythrocyte fragility in exposed patients must be viewed with concern, for increased fragility could result in haemolysis, increasing the level of risk to the fetus. In 1983 Bause *et al*[9] published such a report. Although not statistically significant, they found a trend towards an increase in maternal erythrocyte fragility in patients continuously exposed to Doppler ultrasound monitoring for seven or more hours during labour. The survey was small, involving only 16 patients exposed to ultrasound for periods from one to 29 hours, and eight unexposed controls. The controls differed significantly from the exposed patients in that they spent far shorter periods in labour, less than two hours, compared with 2.75 to 29 hours in the group monitored with Doppler ultrasound. The exposed group was also treated with analgesics which would be expected to dissolve in the plasma membranes of the erythrocytes and affect their permeability. The observed trend towards an increase in erythrocyte fragility in the group exposed to ultrasound could, therefore, have causes other than exposure to Doppler ultrasound, though this cannot be ruled out entirely as a contributory factor.

Advances in *in vitro* fertilisation and implantation techniques in recent years have been accompanied by the use of diagnostic ultrasound to assess follicular growth[10] and to assist in oocyte retrieval[11]. So far little attention has been paid to the effect of this treatment on either the ovary or the released oocytes, although in 1982 there was a report, as yet unconfirmed, of premature ovulation following the use of certain ovulation-inducing medications when ultrasonic scanning was used in the late follicular phase[12]. The clinical significance of this is that oocytes released prematurely are less likely to be successfully fertilised and implanted than those released at maturity. Premature ovulation was observed in 13 out of 41 ultrasonically-scanned patients; of these three followed the use of a real-time scanner, four a static scanner, and six the use of both. No premature ovulation was found in the 24 control patients. It is uncertain, however, if exposure to ultrasound was directly involved in inducing premature ovulation, for the controls were not matched with the exposed patients. Furthermore, the ovaries of the control patients were not subjected to mechanical pressure from a full bladder, as were those of the patients exposed to diagnostic ultrasound, and pressure on the ovary might have been involved in the induction of premature ovulation.

1.2.2 In vivo studies

Most of the investigations in this category have involved the search for increases in the rate of occurrence of developmental abnormalities. Although none has been reported in human populations there have been reports of such increases in small mammals following the use of diagnostic ultrasound. Investigations using small mammals have advantages over human epidemiology in permitting systematic investigation of the mechanisms responsible for the biological effects observed. They have the disadvantage, however, that the results obtained from them are not always directly applicable to the clinical situation.

The work of Shimizu and Shoji[13] and its subsequent analysis by Lele[14] will be considered as an example. Shimizu and Shoji reported an increase in developmental abnormalities in mice exposed to a static scanner for several hours. However, the manner in which the mice were exposed was such that the uterine temperature would be expected to rise to a level sufficient to produce abnormalities even in the absence of ultrasound. Similar temperature increases are unlikely to occur in a pregnant woman, where there is more maternal tissue to attenuate the ultrasound, significantly reducing the intensity to which the fetus is exposed[14]; furthermore, exposure times are considerably shorter. The low temporal average intensities produced by most diagnostic ultrasound instruments also ensure that there is little temperature increase within the target tissues.

Although the temporal average intensities used in diagnostic ultrasound are low (in the mW cm^{-2} range), the temporal peak and pulse average intensities can be much higher (tens of W cm^{-2})[15]. The temporal peak or pulse average intensity may be critically important in affecting the incidence of developmental abnormalities in small mammals, as may their stage of development. In 1981 Takabayashi et al[16] reported that exposure of pregnant mice to a temporal peak intensity of 60 W cm^{-2} was followed by an increase in the incidence of developmental abnormalities, while exposure to 30 W cm^{-2} was not. Both these intensities are within the range of many B-scanners[15], although attenuation by human maternal tissues is far greater than in mice[5, 14], ensuring a considerable reduction in the intensity to which the human embryo or fetus is exposed. The embryos in which an increased incidence of abnormalities was found were at the 8 day stage of intra-uterine development when exposed to ultrasound. This was shown to be a particularly sensitive stage of development, in comparison with the 10 day stage which tolerated higher levels of exposure. Particular caution should, therefore, be observed when exposing early human embryos to ultrasound, in case sensitivity is similarly increased in the early stages of development.

1.2.3 In vitro studies

Many investigations have been carried out in recent years into the effects of ultrasound on mammalian cells maintained in vitro, either in suspension or, less commonly, attached to the surface of culture vessels[17]. Such systems provide the investigator with the opportunity of exploring the mechanisms by which ultrasound can exert effects on individual cells under controlled environmental conditions, but have the disadvantage that the conditions under which the cells are treated may not always apply in vivo, so that extrapolation to the clinical condition is not always appropriate. For example, cavitation, bubble activity induced by ultrasound, is probably responsible for many of the changes produced by ultrasound in vitro. However, the availability of cavitation nuclei may be greater in the culture fluid surrounding cells exposed to ultrasound in vitro than in the extracellular materials by which they are surrounded *in vivo*. There is indirect evidence, obtained from decompression studies and from exposure to therapeutic ultrasound, for the presence of some cavitation nuclei *in vivo*[18], and it has been calculated that in the presence of such nuclei the thresholds for transient cavitation, violent implosion of bubbles resulting in free radical release, are of the order of 10 W cm^{-2} (spatial peak, temporal peak)[19], well within the range used diagnostically. Furthermore, it should be appreciated that cell suspensions are exposed to ultrasound *in vivo* whenever blood, lymph or amniotic fluid, for example, lie in its path, and that the fluid surrounding their cells is rich in dissolved gases and may contain cavitation nuclei.

The biological effects of ultrasound possible *in vitro* which are relevant to its continued safe use *in vivo* include the following:

(a)   inherited changes,
(b)   increased sister chromatid exchange,
(c)   membrane permeability changes.

(a)   Inherited changes
In recent years a major concern in ensuring the continued safe use of ultrasound has been to ensure that exposure to it does not produce an unacceptable increase in changes in inherited characteristics. Although such changes occur naturally, providing the raw materials of evolution, it is generally accepted that most inherited changes are harmful[20]. Many physical and chemical agents to which human populations are exposed increase the rate of inherited change, but exposure to them is considered acceptable because the benefits their use confers far outweigh the risk involved. Should clinical ultrasound fall into this category, then its use would still be permissible provided that the risk was small, for its benefits are so great. Cell cultures provide an excellent means of searching for inherited changes because of the shortness of the cell cycle, i.e. the length of time between successive generations of cells, typically 16 to 24 hours in mammalian cells, and considerably shorter in yeasts and bacteria. In fact, the numerous investigations using such systems have revealed little evidence that exposure to ultrasound at either diagnostic or therapeutic levels does lead to any increase in the frequency of inherited change above that which normally occurs in man[21]. However, further investigations are required to determine the threshold levels for such changes and the mechanisms involved in their production. Should transient cavitation occur, then the free radicals and peroxides generated could have mutagenic effects, as could heat shock, should ultrasound be used at intensities high enough to produce this effect *in vivo* without irreversibly arresting cell division[22].

(b)   Increased sister chromatid exchange
Although there is no conclusive evidence of inherited genetic change as a result of exposure to diagnostic levels of ultrasound *in vitro*[21], there have been some reports of increases in the rate of sister chromatid exchange (SCE). Between 1979 and 1982 at least 14 reports of the effect of ultrasound on SCE were published, of which three were positive[23,24,25].

Sister chromatid exchange occurs during the S and G2 phases of the cell cycle[26], i.e. while the DNA of the chromosomes is being copied (S phase) and in the temporal gap between this and the beginning of mitotic division, when the enzymes needed for cell division are being synthesised. The double-stranded helical DNA of each chromosome copies itself exactly, utilising specific base pairing to do so, each original chromosome together with its newly-produced duplicate forming a pair of sister chromatids. Sometimes while the two components of each sister chromatid pair are still in apposition genetic recombination occurs. The two homologous double-stranded DNA helices, one longitudinally arranged in each sister chromatid, break, and the resulting DNA fragments are exchanged before the breaks are repaired. The site of the exchange may be anywhere along the length of the homologous nucleotide sequences which comprise the DNA of each chromatid pair. At the site of exchange, a staggered joint, typically thousands of base-pairs long, is formed between the DNA helices of the two adjacent sister chromatids. No nucleotide sequences are altered at the place of exchange, the breaking and reunion being so precisely controlled that not a single nucleotide is lost, gained or substituted, the staggering of the joints ensuring that only identical, homologous regions of DNA are exchanged. Because the chromatids in each pair are identical, the exchange does not produce inherited changes.

The genetic recombination involved in SCE can only take place if breaks occur in each of the double strands of DNA of the two adjacent sister chromatids of a single chromatid pair, freeing homologous fragments of the DNA strands for the helical unwinding, mutual exchange and rewinding events required. A single break in one of the strands is all that is needed to initiate recombination, the other breaks developing in response to this in a controlled manner, resulting, after exchange, in perfect repair. Although SCE may be a normal occurrence, agents known to introduce breaks in DNA strands, for example γ- and X-irradiation, can increase its rate. Since after exchange the two sister chromatids are genetically identical, the exchanges cannot be detected by genetic means. They can, however, be visualised during the metaphase stage of mitosis either by autoradiography[27] or by the application of a specific staining technique[28]. In the autoradiographic procedure the cells are allowed one replication cycle in culture medium containing ^{3}H-thymidine, followed by a second cycle in medium containing unlabelled thymidine. At the second metaphase only one chromatid of each pair contains radiolabelled thymidine, unless SCE has occurred, when the label switches between the chromatids at one or more points along their length. Each switch represents an instance of SCE exchange. In the staining procedure the cells must first be grown in the presence of the thymidine analogue 5-bromo-2′-deoxyuridine (BrdU). BrdU is readily incorporated into DNA during synthesis, in place of thymidine, from which it differs only in that it has a bromine atom at the position of a methyl group. A specific staining technique, generally referred to as "fluorescence plus Giemsa"[28], stains thymidine-containing DNA more intensely than that containing BrdU. If SCE occurs, this differential staining causes the chromatids to take on a striped appearance, the stripes of one member of each chromatid pair being the reciprocal of those of the other. The number of stripes on each harlequin-like chromatid is equivalent to the number of exchanges that have occurred during one cell cycle.

Although the biological significance of SCE is uncertain[29], it has been suggested[26] that the close, though temporary, proximity of the DNA strands during the S and G2 phases of the cell cycle may allow for controlled repair of DNA damage, the undamaged strands acting as templates for the others, so that perfect repair is possible. Increase in SCE could, therefore, indicate that although damage, in the form of an increased number of DNA breaks, has occurred, the damage has been corrected without genetic change. Whether or not SCE occurs spontaneously is a matter of conjecture, for the agents used to detect it (^{3}H-thymidine and BrdU) are themselves capable of inducing it, and will remain unresolved until innocuous detection procedures have been developed.

The majority of studies of the effect of diagnostic ultrasound on SCE have yielded negative results[30] but the consistently positive findings described by Liebeskind[23], Haupt[24] and Ehlinger[25] and their colleagues give cause for concern and require both critical assessment and confirmation. Major difficulties in comparing the results obtained by different groups are the wide variation in frequency, intensity, exposure times and exposure methods used, and valid comparisons cannot be made until standardised irradiation procedures are adopted. A feature of biological, and possibly clinical, significance is that there is variation in the susceptibility of different cell types to the induction of SCE when similar irradiation procedures are used; thus Liebeskind found an increase in SCE in human lymphoctes[23], but not in HeLa cells[31], even when the latter were exposed to higher intensities of ultrasound. In the light of this the possibility of variation in sensitivity of different cell types at different stages of development requires investigation.

One of the reasons that the demonstration of increase in SCE following treatment with any physical or chemical agent gives rise to concern is that a positive linear relationship has been demonstrated between such exchanges and both *in vitro* cell transformation[32] and carcinogenicity, SCE analysis being 80 per cent to 90 per cent predictive[33, 34]. However, as with all short term tests, SCE analysis is subject to both false positives and false negatives, and as far as ultrasound is concerned, no connection has been found between exposure to diagnostic ultrasound and the incidence of cancer[34, 35].

(c) Membrane permeability changes
Although there is little evidence that exposure to diagnostic levels of ultrasound can induce genetic changes[37], there are indications that the levels used therapeutically can affect cell behaviour via changes to the cell membrane. Should similar membrane-mediated effects occur during embryogenesis, then its outcome could be affected. Since therapeutic and diagnostic levels overlap (see *table 1.1*) it is in the interests of the continued safe use of ultrasound that the thresholds for these effects, and the mechanisms inducing them, be determined.

Exposure to ultrasound has been shown to affect the transport of ions and molecules across cell membranes. For example, Chapman[38] demonstrated a decreased influx and increased efflux of potassium ions in thymocytes following exposure to 0.5–3.0 MHz CW ultrasound at spatial average, temporal average intensities of 0.4–3.0 W cm^{-2}. Changes have also been observed in the calcium ion concentration within fibroblasts[39] and in the uptake of ^{3}H-leucine in avian erythrocytes after exposure to ultrasound at levels within the therapeutic range[40]. All the above changes were obtained following *in vitro* treatment of cell suspensions with ultrasound in conditions in which cavitation could readily occur. The permeability changes were not associated with cell lysis, and it is likely that they, and many of the other changes reported in cell surface morphology and function[3], are related to shear forces established by ultrasonically-mediated fluid flow, possibly associated with cavitation[41]. Modification of the permeability of the cell surface to, for example, calcium ions, can have far-reaching effects on cell behaviour, resulting in a wide variety of changes, including increased synthesis of protein[42], increased secretion [43, 44, 45] and motility changes[31, 39]. Although such effects can be of therapeutic value[3], they could have undesirable effects on

7

embryogenesis, and every effort should be made to minimise them when ultrasound is used diagnostically, particularly during early pregnancy.

1.3 Conclusions

If the mechanisms and thresholds involved in the production of potentially hazardous biological effects by ultrasound are known, then diagnostic ultrasound can be used in such a manner that these effects are avoided. Many have a thermal origin, and are unlikely to result from the obstetric use of diagnostic ultrasound as it is currently applied, because the spatial average, temporal average intensities produced are too low to produce significant heating of the target, the embryo or fetus, particularly when attenuation by the maternal tissues is taken into consideration.

There is less cause for complacency with regard to cavitation, for it has been shown theoretically[19] that if appropriate nuclei are present, potentially damaging transient cavitation can be induced by microsecond pulses of ultrasound at diagnostic intensities. This has now been demonstrated practically in fluids[46]. The conditions required for transient cavitation *in vivo* are peak intensities at the target site of 2–50 W cm^{-2} depending on the frequency[19] and the existence of cavitation nuclei. Many pulse echo units currently in use exceed these outputs[47], although the input to the target site is generally much lower than the output because of attenuation by the maternal tissues. There is indirect evidence for the presence of cavitation nuclei *in vivo*, but so far no clear evidence to support the possibility that cavitation may affect the fetus[47]. However, there has been little adequately controlled work on the effects of ultrasound, either cavitational or thermal, on early developmental processes, some of which may have a reduced threshold of sensitivity to environmental changes. Until more is known of the distribution of cavitation nuclei in and around developing tissues, caution is advised in the use of diagnostic ultrasound at levels above the threshold for transient cavitation in the presence of such nuclei. These thresholds are of the order of 10 W cm^{-2}, (spatial peak, temporal peak)[47]. According to Carstensen and Gates[47] almost all the diagnostic procedures used in obstetrics can be performed with peak intensities well below this level.

The continued safe use of diagnostic ultrasound, particularly as it is applied in obstetrics, would be ensured more readily if information on the peak output of all diagnostic ultrasound generators were available to their operators, and if, in line with the recent recommendations of the National Council for Radiation Protection and Measurements, the exposure of the patient to diagnostic ultrasound was minimised, within the limits of obtaining the necessary diagnostic information[1]. The benefits conferred by the proper use of diagnostic ultrasound are far too valuable for them to be jeopardised by its abuse.

Acknowledgements
I wish to thank Mr S R Young, Ms M Harrison and Mrs R Hickman for their technical assistance, and the National Fund for Research into Crippling Diseases (Action Research) for support (grant number A/8/1153).

References

1 NATIONAL COUNCIL ON RADIATION PROTECTION AND MEASUREMENTS 1983 *Biological effects of ultrasound: mechanisms and clinical implications* Report 74 (NCRP Publications, 7910 Woodmont Avenue, Bethesda, MD 20814, USA)

2 NYBORG W L and ZISKIN M C 1985 (eds) *Biological Effects of Ultrasound* Vol **16** *Clinics in Diagnostic Ultrasound* (Churchill Livingstone Inc: New York)

3 DYSON M 1985 Therapeutic applications of ultrasound In: *Biological effects of ultrasound* Nyborg W L and Ziskin M C (Eds) Vol **16** *Clinics in Diagnostic Ultrasound* pp 121–123 (Churchill Livingstone Inc: New York)

4 DYSON M 1982 Non-thermal cellular effects of ultrasound *British Journal of Cancer* **45** (Suppl V) 165–171

5 LELE P P 1979 Revue: safety and potential hazards in the current applications of ultrasound in obstetrics and gynecology *Ultrasound in Medicine and Biology* **5** 307–320

6 ENVIRONMENTAL HEALTH DIRECTORATE 1980 *Canada-wide survey of nonionizing radiation emitting devices Part II Ultrasound devices* Report 80–EHD–53 (Environmental Health Directorate, Health Protection Branch: Ottawa)

7 MOORE R M Jr, BARRICK K M and HAMILTON T M 1982 Effect of sonic radiation on growth and development *Proceedings of the Meeting of the Society for Epidemiological Research* Cincinnati Ohio June 16–18

8 STARK C R, ORLEANS M, HAVERKAMP A D and MURPHY J 1984 Short- and long-term risks after exposure to diagnostic ultrasound in utero *Obstetrics and Gynecology* **63** 194–200

9 BAUSE G S, NIEBYL J R and SANDERS R C 1983 Doppler Ultrasound and Maternal Erythrocyte Fragility *Obstetrics and Gynecology* **62** 7–10

10 KERIN J F, EDMOND D K, WARNES G M, COX L W, SEAMARK R F, MATTHEWS C D, YOUNG G B and BAIRD D T 1981 Morphological and functional relations of Graafian follicle growth to ovulation in women using ultrasonic, laparascopic and biochemical measurements *British Journal of Obstetrics and Gynaecology* **88** 81–90

11 LENZ S, LAURITSEN J G and KJELLOW M 1981 Collection of human oocytes for in vitro fertilisation by ultrasonically guided follicular puncture *Lancet* **i** 1163–1164

12 TESTART J, INSERM U, THEBAULT A, SOUDERES E and FRYDMAN R 1982 Premature ovulation after ovarian ultrasonography *British Journal of Obstetrics and Gynaecology* **89** 694–700

13 SHIMIZU T and SHOJI R 1973 An experimental safety study of mice exposed to low intensity ultrasound In: *Proceedings of the Second World Congress on Ultrasonics in Medicine* de Vleiger M, White D N and McCready V R (Eds) Excerpta Medica Inter-National Congress Series No 277 (Excerpta Medica Foundation: Amsterdam) p 28

14 LELE P P 1975 Ultrasonic teratology in mouse and man In: *Proceedings of the Second European Congress on Ultrasonics in Medicine* Kazner E, de Vleiger M, Muller H R and McCready V R (Eds) Excerpta Medica International Congress Series No 363 (Excerpta Medica Foundation: Amsterdam) p 22

15 NYBORG W L 1985 Mechanisms In: *Biological Effects of Ultrasound* Nyborg W L and Ziskin M C (Eds) Vol **16** *Clinics in Diagnostic Ultrasound* pp 23–34 (Churchill Livingstone Inc: New York)

16 TAKABAYASHI T, ABE T, SATO S and SUZUKI M 1981 Study of pulsewave ultrasonic irradiation on mouse embryos *Cho'onpa Igaku (Medical Ultrasound)* **8** 286

17 SIEGEL E, GODDARD J, JAMES A E Jr and SIEGEL E P 1979 Cellular attachment as a sensitive indicator of the effects of diagnostic ultrasound exposure on cultured human cells *Radiology* **133** 175–179

18 TER HAAR G and DANIELS S 1981 Evidence of ultrasonically induced cavitation in vivo *Physics in Medicine and Biology* **26** 1145–1150

19 FLYNN H G 1982 Generation of transient cavities in liquids by microsecond pulses of ultrasound *Journal of the Acoustical Society of America* **72** 1926–1931

20 EDWARDS J H 1979 The cost of mutation In: *Genetic Damage in man Caused by Environmental Agents* Berg K (Ed) p 465 (Academic Press: New York)

21 THACKER J 1985 Investigations into Genetic and Inherited Changes Produced by Ultrasound In: *Biological Effects of Ultrasound* Nyborg W L and Ziskin M C (eds) pp 67–76 (Churchill Livingstone Inc: New York)

22 THACKER J 1973 The possibility of genetic hazard from ultrasonic irradiation *Current Topics in Radiation Research* **8** 235

23 LIEBESKIND D, BASES R, MENDEZ F, ELEQUIN F and KOENIGSBERG M 1979 Sister chromatid exchanges in human lymphocytes after exposure to diagnostic ultrasound *Science* **205** 1273–1275

24 HAUPT M, MARTIN A O, SIMPSON J L, IQBAL M A, ELIAS S, DYER A and SABBAGHA R E 1981 Ultrasonic induction of sister chromatid exchanges in human lymphocytes *Human Genetics* **59** 221–226

25 EHLINGER C A, KATAYAMA K P, ROELER M R and MATTINGLY R F 1981 Diagnostic ultrasound increases sister chromatid exchange, preliminary report *Wisconsin Medical Journal* **80** 21–22

26 ALBERTS B, BRAY D, LEWIS J, RAFF M, ROBERTS K and WATSON J D 1983 *Molecular Biology of the Cell* (Garland Publishing Inc: New York)

27 TAYLOR J H 1958 Sister chromatid exchange in tritium labelled chromosomes *Genetics* **43** 515

28 WOLFF S and PERRY P 1974 Differential Giemsa staining of sister chromatids and the study of sister chromatid exchange without autoradiography *Chromosoma* **48** 341–353

29 JACOBSON-KRAM D 1984 The effects of diagnostic ultrasound on sister chromatid exchange frequencies *Journal of Clinical Ultrasound* **12** 5–10

30 MILLER M W 1985 In Vitro Studies: Single Cells and Multicell Spheroids In: *Biological Effects of Ultrasound* Nyborg W L and Ziskin M C (Eds) Vol **16** *Clinics in Diagnostic Ultrasound* (Churchill Livingstone Inc: New York)

31 LIEBESKIND D, BASES R, KOENIGSBERG M, KOSS L and RAVENTOS C 1981 Morphological changes in the surface characteristics of cultured cells after exposure to diagnostic ultrasound *Radiology* **138** 419–423

32 POPESCU N C, AMSBAUGH S C, DiPAOLO J A 1981 Relationship of carcinogen-induced sister chromatid exchange and neoplastic cell transformation *International Journal of Cancer* **28** 71–77

33 LATT S A, ALLEN J, BLOOM S et al 1981 Sister chromatid exchanges: A report of the GENE-TOX program *Mutation Research* **87** 17–62

34 ABE S and SASAKI M 1982 In: *Sister Chromatid Exchange* Sandberg A A (Ed) pp 461–514 (Alan R Liss: New York)

35 KINNIER WILSON L M and WATERHOUSE J A H 1984 Obstetric ultrasound and childhood malignancies *Lancet* **ii** 997–999

36 CARTWRIGHT R A, McKINNEY P A, HOPTON P A, BIRCH J M, HARTLEY A L, MANN J R, WATERHOUSE J A H, JOHNSTON H E, DRAPER G J and STILLER C 1984 Ultrasound examinations in pregnancy and childhood cancer *Lancet* **ii** 999–1000

37 MARTIN A 1984 Can ultrasound cause genetic damage? *Journal of Clinical Ultrasound* **12** 11–20

38 CHAPMAN I V, MacNALLY N A and TUCKER S 1979 Ultrasound induced changes in rates of influx and efflux of potassium ions in rat thymocytes in vitro *Ultrasound in Medicine and Biology* **6** 47–58

39 MUMMERY C L 1978 *The effect of ultrasound on fibroblasts in vitro* PhD Thesis, University of London

40 BUNDY M L, LERNER J, MESSIER D L and ROONEY J A 1978 Effects of ultrasound on transport in avian erythrocytes *Ultrasound in Medicine and Biology* **4** 259–262

41 DOULAH M S 1977 Mechanism of disintegration of biological cells in ultrasonic cavitation *Biotechnology and Bioengineering* **19** 649

10

42   WEBSTER D F, POND J B, DYSON M and HARVEY W 1978 The role of cavitation in the in vitro stimulation of protein synthesis in human fibroblasts by ultrasound *Ultrasound in Medicine and Biology* **4** 343–351

43   FYFE M C and CHAHL L A 1984 Mast cell degranulation and increased vascular permeability induced by 'therapeutic' ultrasound in the rat ankle joint *British Journal of Experimental Pathology* **65** 671–676

44   HASHISH I and HARVEY W 1985 Degranulation of mast cells by therapeutic ultrasound *Journal of Dental Research* **64** 670

45   DYSON M and LUKE D A 1986 Induction of Mast Cell Degranulation in Skin by Ultrasound IEEE UFFC, **33** 194–201

46   CRUM L A and FOWLKES J B 1986 Acoustic cavitation generated by microsecond pulses of ultrasound *Nature* **319** 52–54

47   CARSTENSEN E L and GATES A H 1985 Ultrasound and the Mammalian Fetus In: *Biological Effects of Ultrasound* Nyborg W L and Ziskin M C (Eds) Vol **16** *Clinics in Diagnostic Ultrasound* pp 85–96 (Churchill Livingstone Inc: New York)

CHAPTER 2

Wave Propagation in Tissues

J A Evans
Department of Medical Physics, University of Leeds, Leeds General Infirmary, Leeds LS1 3EX

2.1 Attenuation in tissue

As a compressional ultrasound wave passes through biological tissue or any similar material, it will be subject to attenuation due to a variety of processes. The major mechanisms of attenuation are normally accepted to be:

(a) Beam spreading due to diffraction as a result of using finite sources and receivers.

(b) Reflections at large ($>> \lambda$) interfaces between regions of differing acoustic impedance.

(c) Scattering at small ($<< \lambda$) interfaces which accounts for much of the diagnostic information commonly used.

(d) Mode conversion at soft-hard tissue interfaces, where shear wave generation can occur.

(e) Absorption processes by which acoustic energy is converted directly to heat.

(f) Non-linear effects which cause the generation of high frequency components and shock-waves.

(g) Cavitational losses due to energy dissipation associated with small bubbles in the system.

It is clearly impossible to deal adequately with all of these processes in the available space and so attention will be necessarily focussed on one or two small aspects of the whole problem. It is generally assumed that the cavitational losses (g) are not likely to be significant for low intensity, short, diagnostic pulses and thus they will not be discussed further. The losses due to diffraction (a) are strongly dependent upon the nature of the source rather than the tissue itself and so will also be eliminated from further discussion. Non-linear effects (f) are discussed at some length elsewhere in this book and so will not be treated here. The remaining processes reflection (b), scattering (c), mode conversion (d) and absorption (e) are clearly tissue specific and merit closer examination.

It is possible to attempt to evaluate the relative contribution of each process to the total observed attenuation. A distinction must first be drawn between losses such as reflection and mode conversion which are associated with boundaries between tissue types, and absorption and scattering which occur during the propagation of the pulse through a single tissue. Wells[1] has summarised some of the tissue-specific data and this is reproduced in *figure 2.1*.

It can readily be seen from *figure 2.1* that the attenuation values for soft tissues are substantial and for that reason the remainder of this discussion will be devoted to consideration of propagation through single tissue regions. It can also be seen that the attenuation due to a typical, soluble, globular protein, haemoglobin, is

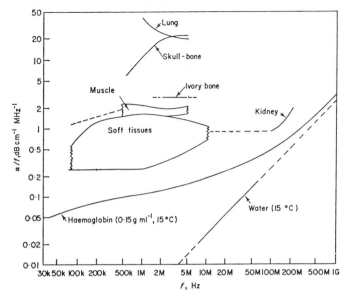

Figure 2.1 Compilation of tissue attenuation data (after Wells[1]).

almost as large as that of many soft tissues in the 1–10 MHz range. Indeed, studies on proteins in solution generally have produced similar values[2].

However, as Goss *et al*[3] have reported, the data on the 'building blocks' of these proteins, amino acids, have generally resulted in very low values of absorption, roughly comparable with pure water.

Attempts have been made to investigate this more fully. Pauly and Schwan[4] measured the attenuation of beef and lamb liver which they then proceeded to homogenise. In the homogenisation process the cellular structure was destroyed and yet the attenuation value dropped only slightly (about 20 per cent). The absorption coefficient of the fluid in the homogenate was found to be similar to that of haemoglobin. Thus it was concluded that most of the attenuation occurred at a macromolecular rather than cellular level and that the scattering contribution was small relative to the true absorption. It is therefore important to develop a theory which satisfactorily explains both the magnitude and the frequency dependence of the absorption coefficient of macromolecular solutions.

2.2 Absorption mechanisms

Traditionally, the absorption of acoustic energy by fluids has been attributed to mechanisms categorised as either 'classical' or 'non-classical'[5]. Although there is some inconsistency in the literature, it is normally the case that the classical contribution is taken to be a combination of the shear viscosity losses first described by Stokes[6] and losses due to heat conduction in the medium[7]. The shear viscosity process leads to absorption described by

$$\alpha = \frac{2}{3} \frac{\eta}{\kappa} \frac{\omega^2}{c} \tag{1}$$

13

where α is the absorption coefficient, η is the viscosity, κ is the bulk modulus of elasticity, ω is the angular frequency and c is the velocity.

It is clear from the above equation that the Stokes model predicts that α will be proportional to the square of the frequency which is not consistent with experimental data on biological liquids. Further, if reasonable values are substituted into the equation the predicted value of α at low MHz frequencies is roughly two orders of magnitude smaller than the observed values. However, it should be noted that the Stokes model provides a much more accurate description of the acoustic behaviour of pure water.

The Kirchoff heat conduction model is generally accepted not to produce a significant contribution in the biological fluids and so the total 'classical' contribution remains very small.

All other postulated mechanisms are conventionally described as 'non-classical' and all involve relaxation processes. Of these mechanisms, the most relevant are those which are sometimes collectively described as contributing a 'volume viscosity' term. These can be further subdivided but it is instructive to first examine the general underlying theory of relaxation. In order to do this, it is necessary to consider the general equations of wave propagation as they apply to biological fluids.

2.3   Wave propagation equations

In general, the simplest expression for a wave propagating in one-dimension is the wave equation in terms of some parameter ϕ

$$\frac{\delta^2 \phi}{\delta x^2} = \frac{1}{c^2}\frac{\delta^2 \phi}{\delta t^2} \tag{2}$$

where c is the wave velocity, t is the time and x is the direction of propagation.

This has the general solution

$$\phi = \phi_0\, e^{i2\pi(ft-\beta x)} \tag{3}$$

where $\beta = \dfrac{1}{\lambda}$ is the wavenumber and f is the frequency.

If absorption is present, this becomes

$$\phi = \phi_0 = e^{i2\pi(ft-\beta x)}e^{-\alpha x} \tag{4}$$

If ϕ is taken to be the amplitude of the wave, then α is the amplitude absorption coefficient.

It is possible to re-arrange this into

$$\phi = \phi_0\, e^{i2\pi(ft-\gamma^* x)} \tag{5}$$

where $\gamma^* = \beta - \dfrac{i\alpha}{2\pi}$, is a complex quantity. This would imply a complex velocity c^*, given by

$$c^* = \frac{f}{\gamma^*} \tag{6}$$

14

Before proceeding further, it should be noted that the above equations apply to any one-dimensional wave and therefore the analogy between acoustic and electromagnetic waves can be pursued, as in *table 2.1*. One interesting aspect of the data of *table 2.1* is the correspondence between the permittivity of the medium for electromagnetic waves and the compressibility for acoustic waves. These results are important when trying to apply knowledge of mechanisms gleaned from r.f. studies to the ultrasound case. They also demonstrate that if the real and imaginary parts of the compressibility are known then the medium is completely characterised and values of α and c can be computed from them.

Table 2.1 Analogy between electromagnetic and acoustic wave propagation.

Electromagnetic Waves	Acoustic Waves
$$c^2 = \frac{1}{\epsilon^* \mu}$$	$$c^2 = \frac{1}{\kappa^* \rho}$$
where ϵ^*-permittivity, μ-permeability	where $\kappa^* = $ compressibility, $\rho = $ density
Assume $\mu = \mu_0 = $ constant	Assume $\rho = \rho_0 = $ constant
Then $\epsilon^* = \epsilon' - i\,\epsilon''$	Then $\kappa^* = \kappa' - i\,\kappa''$
But $\gamma = \beta - \dfrac{\alpha}{2\pi}$	But $\gamma = \beta - \dfrac{\alpha}{2\pi}$
and $(c^*)^2 = f^2/(\gamma^*)^2$	and $(c^*)^2 = f^2/(\gamma^*)^2$
Comparing real and imaginary parts gives:	
$$\epsilon' = \frac{1}{\mu_0 \omega^2}[(2\pi\beta)^2 - \alpha^2]$$	$$\kappa' = \frac{1}{\rho_0 \omega^2}[(2\pi\beta)^2 - \alpha^2]$$
and	
$$\epsilon'' = \frac{4\pi}{\mu_0 \omega^2}\alpha\beta$$	$$\kappa'' = \frac{4\pi}{\rho_0 \omega^2}\alpha\beta$$

2.4 Relaxation theory

In order to apply the knowledge of the propagation equations to biological systems, it is necessary to formulate the relaxation mechanisms.

In general, for any relaxing system with a thermodynamic parameter $Y = Y(X, q)$,

$$\frac{dY}{dX} = \left(\frac{\delta Y}{\delta X}\right)_\infty + \left[\left(\frac{\delta Y}{\delta X}\right)_0 - \left(\frac{\delta Y}{\delta X}\right)_\infty\right]\left(\frac{1 - i\omega\tau}{1 + \omega^2\tau^2}\right) \quad (7)$$

where τ is the relaxation time, and the subscripts ∞ and o refer to infinite and zero frequency.

15

For example, if $X = \dfrac{1}{\rho} \dfrac{\delta\rho}{\delta p}$ (8)

at constant entropy, then

$$Y = p, x = p \text{ and } \kappa^* = q \tag{9}$$

Then

$$\kappa^* = \kappa_\infty + (\kappa_0 - \kappa_\infty) \frac{1 - i\,\omega\tau}{1 + \omega^2\,\tau^2} \tag{10}$$

and it can be shown that

$$\kappa' = \kappa_\infty + \frac{\kappa_0 - \kappa_\infty}{1 + \omega^2\,\tau^2} \tag{11}$$

and

$$\kappa'' = \frac{(\kappa_0 - \kappa_\infty)\,\omega\tau}{1 + \omega^2\,\tau^2} \tag{12}$$

Thus by measuring κ' and κ'' over the frequency range of interest, the relaxation process can be fully characterised. It is also important to realise that the imaginary quantity κ'' corresponds closely to the quantity $\alpha\,\lambda$ which is frequently quoted in the literature (see *table 2.1*). For typical cases in the medical frequency range, κ' will be very much greater than κ'' and the contribution of the $(\alpha)^2$ term to the value κ' (*table 2.1*) will be small and hence the velocity dispersions will normally be small also.

2.5 Specific relaxation processes

It should be noted that equation (8) is valid only for constant entropy situations. This corresponds to a system at equilibrium in which the pressure change associated with the ultrasound wave causes a volume change and an associated equilibrium position shift. It is also possible to analyse the system at constant volume in which case it is the temperature rise associated with the wave which causes the shift in equilibrium. These two cases are sometimes described as thermal (i.e. temperature sensitive) and non-thermal (i.e. pressure sensitive) relaxation mechanisms.

The two best known thermal mechanisms are vibrational and isomeric relaxations. Space does not permit these cases to be evaluated here but they can be shown to be negligible for most biological fluids. Thus the options are finally limited to non-thermal mechanisms involving pressure sensitive equilibria with the associated volume changes. These are sometimes referred to as structural relaxations.

One such relaxation is well-known and has been widely studied. It involves so-called proton-transfer equilibria at protein side-chains. Either the carboxyl or amino groups can be involved depending upon pH. Thus,

16

$$\text{Acid pH} \qquad\qquad \text{Neutral pH} \qquad\qquad \text{Alkaline pH}$$

$$R\begin{array}{c}\nearrow NH_3\\ \searrow COOH\end{array} + OH^- \rightleftharpoons R\begin{array}{c}\nearrow NH_3{}^+\\ \searrow COO^-\end{array} + H_2O \rightleftharpoons R\begin{array}{c}\nearrow NH_2\\ \searrow COO^-\end{array} + H_3O^+$$

Thus a proton can be attached to either side group or transferred to the bulk water molecules.

That these reactions can be significant was well demonstrated by Kessler and Dunn[8] who found increases of up to 50 per cent in the absorption of a soluble protein (*figure 2.2*), bovine serum albumin when the pH of the solution was changed. Since then pH-related changes have been found in many biological solutions including amino acids.

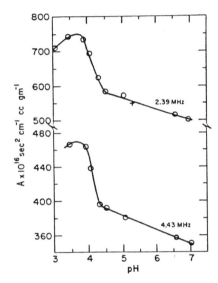

Figure 2.2   Absorption of BSA as a function of pH (after Kessler and Dunn[8]).

Other workers have suggested different structural relaxations might be significant at neutral pH. Helix-random coil transition equilibria have been suggested as well as rather vague notions of solute-solvent reactions. None of these has been convincingly shown to contribute significantly at neutral pH.

However, a significant step forward was made by Slutsky *et al*[9] who directed attention to the imidazole ring of the histidyl residue which is to be found in many proteins. This residue can participate in a proton-transfer reaction with phosphate ions in solution and is at equilibrium close to neutral pH. The presence of the phosphate ion in the surrounding solution can increase the absorption by over 100 per cent at 2 MHz (*figure 2.3*). Generalising these results to the *in-vivo* case of protein with N such sites, Slutsky *et al*[10] estimated the contribution to tissue absorption by this mechanism alone and produced figures which were almost equal to observed values.

17

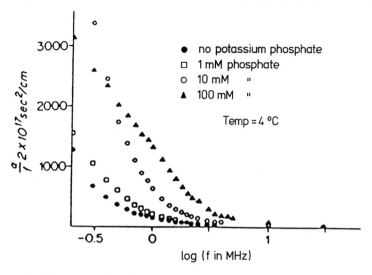

Figure 2.3 Absorption of Bacitracin as a function of frequency and phosphate ion concentration (after Slutsky *et al*[9]).

The imidazole-phosphate model rests upon several major assumptions of which the most critical is perhaps that the total protein absorption is the sum of its constituent amino-acid residue absorptions. This is almost certainly not true since amino acids in proteins find themselves in complex three-dimensional structures in which the local environment may be quite different from that of bulk free water[11]. Nevertheless, this work represents a significant step forward in our understanding.

We thus have a situation in which a single type of process, proton-transfer equilibria perturbation, has emerged as likely to provide the dominant contribution to ultrasonic absorption in protein solutions and probably, tissue. Much more work remains to be done before this can finally be established but in the meantime it may be worthwhile to examine the clinical implications. These are not at all clear but if absorption is taking place at preferred sites, i.e. sites of proton-transfer, then it is possible that these will be particularly sensitive to ultrasound and investigators concerned with ultrasound safety may wish to consider this. Secondly, workers who are concerned with precise measurement of attenuation in tissue may wish to take extra care that environmental factors such as pH, phosphate ion concentration and temperature are well controlled and recorded. Whether any further direct clinical application stems from this improved understanding will emerge in the near future.

Acknowledgements

The author would like to gratefully acknowledge the help of Dr C Barnes and Professor T J Lewis in the preparation of this paper.

References

1 WELLS P N T 1977 *Biomedical Ultrasonics* (Academic Press, London)
2 KREMKAU F W and COWGILL R W 1985 Biomolecular Absorption of Ultrasound: II Molecular Structure *J Acoust Soc Am* **77**(3) 1217–1221
3 GOSS S A, JOHNSTON R L, MAYNARD V, DERL N, FRIZZELL L A, O'BRIEN W D Jnr and DUNN F 1979 *Ultrasonic Tissue Characterisation II* NBS Spec Pub 525 (Edited by M Linzer) US Govt Printing Office
4 PAULY H and SCHWAN H P 1971 Mechanism of absorption of ultrasound in liver tissue *J Acoust Soc Am* **50**(2) 692–699
5 MARKHAM J J, BEYER R T and LINDSAY R B 1951 Absorption of sound in fluids *Rev Mod Phys* **23**(4) 353–411
6 STOKES GG 1845 On the theories of the internal friction of fluids in motion and of the equilibrium and motion of elastic solids *Trans Cambridge Phil Soc* **8** 287–319
7 KIRCHOFF G 1868 Ueber den Einflufs der Wörmebitung in einem Gase auf die Schallbewegung *Annalen Der Physik Und Chemie* **134** 177–193
8 KESSLER L W and DUNN F 1969 Ultrasonic investigation of the conformal changes of bovine serum albumin in aqueous solution *J Phys Chem* **73** 4256–4263
9 SLUTSKY L J, MADSEN L, WHITE R D and HARKNESS J 1980 Kinetics of the exchange of protons between hydrogen phosphate ions and a histidyl residue *J Phys Chem* **84** 1325–1329
10 SLUTSKY L J 1981 Ultrasonic chemical relaxation spectroscopy — Chapter 4 in *Methods In Experimental Physics Vol 19* (Edited by P D Edmonds) (Academic Press, London)
11 PETHIG R 1979 *Dielectric and Electronic Properties of Biological Materials* (J Wiley and Sons, London)

CHAPTER 3

Portable Equipment and Techniques for Measurement of Ultrasonic Power and Intensity

K Martin
Regional Medical Physics Department, Newcastle General Hospital, Newcastle-upon-Tyne NE4 6BE

3.1 Introduction

Following recent publicity about the possibility of adverse biological effects due to exposure to diagnostic ultrasound, especially in the case of obstetric investigations, there has been an increased demand for knowledge of the acoustic output power and intensity of ultrasound equipment. Although some manufacturers will provide such information for customers, it is preferable to make independent measurements on each machine in use as manufacturers may provide only typical values for each model of scanner and transducer. Thus the hospital physicist may be required to visit a remote hospital and make a comprehensive range of acoustic power and intensity measurements on a scanning machine with a range of transducers.

The most widely accepted measurement standards and procedures are described in the AIUM/NEMA Standards Publication No. UL1–1981[1]. This standard requires manufacturers of diagnostic ultrasound equipment to provide measurements of ultrasonic power, spatial peak-temporal average intensity (I_{SPTA}), spatial peak-pulse average intensity (I_{SPPA}) and spatial average-temporal average intensity (I_{SATA}). Some of the measurement procedures recommended in this standard are difficult and time consuming using simple, portable test equipment. In particular, measurement of I_{SPTA} for real time scanning machines may require internal triggering signals, detailed knowledge of the scanning sequence and the capture and integration of a large number of ultrasonic pulses. As I_{SPTA} is the acoustic intensity parameter referred to in the AIUM Bioeffects committee statement on the biological effects of ultrasound in mammalian tissue, it is also likely to be the parameter of most interest.

This paper is a description of the equipment and techniques used by the author to make field measurements of the power and intensity parameters above following the requirements of *reference 1* as closely as possible.

3.2 Equipment

The portable equipment used to make acoustic power and intensity measurements is illustrated in *figure 3.1* and consists of the following:

1. Portable radiation force balance.
2. Calibrated PVDF bilaminar hydrophone with 1 mm diameter active element.
3. Hydrophone preamplifier.
4. 2 gallon bucket with 3 axis micromanipulator and mounting plate.

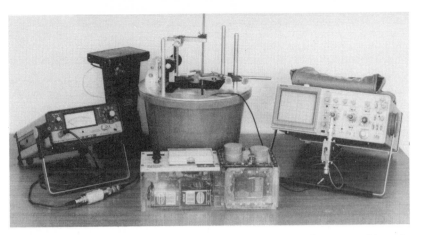

Figure 3.1 Assembled portable equipment used to make acoustic power and intensity measurements.

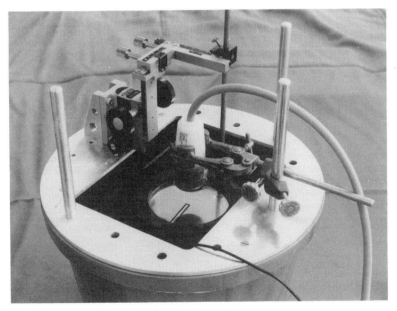

Figure 3.2 The micromanipulator and hydrophone assembly used for acoustic intensity measurements.

5. Modified portable oscilloscope.
6. Polaroid camera.
7. R.f. power meter with thermocouple sensor.
(see appendix for further details of equipment)

For intensity measurements, the bucket is filled with tap water and the hydrophone is suspended in the water from the micromanipulator via a 6 mm rod and clamp (see *figure 3.2*). The transducer under test is mounted with retort clamps so that the ultrasonic beam propagates vertically downwards into the water. A piece of carpet is placed on the bottom of the bucket to reduce reflections. Hydrophone signals are displayed on the oscilloscope via the hydrophone preamplifier.

3.3 Measurement techniques

3.3.1 Ultrasonic power

The total ultrasonic power output from diagnostic ultrasound machines is most conveniently measured using a portable radiation force balance. Currently, there appears to be only one such instrument available commercially (Model UMR.4 from SIEL, Unit 8, Young's Industrial Estate, Paice's Hill, Aldermaston, Berks) but designs suitable for construction in Medical Physics Departments, have been described in the literature[2,3]. The instrument used by the author is a water filled version of that described by Farmery and Whittingham[2]. This balance may be used to make ultrasonic power measurements over the range 0.5 mW to 100 mW.

The projection of the length of the absorbing target in the force balance onto the acoustic window against which the transducer is placed is 2.7 cm. Thus measurements can be made conveniently on single element transducers and sector scanner transducers operated in M-mode. In the case of linear arrays however, it is necessary to estimate the total power output by arranging the array so that it overlaps the whole width of the target and then multiplying the power reading by L/2.7 where L cm is the active length of the array.

Scanning machine controls are set to give maximum power for each machine/ transducer combination.

3.3.2 Spatial peak temporal average intensity (I_{SPTA})

(a) Theory
The spatial peak temporal average intensity is the temporal average intensity at the point in the acoustic field where the temporal average intensity is a maximum. For real time imaging systems, the temporal average is taken over one or more complete scan repetition periods whereas for other systems the average is taken over one or more pulse repetition periods.

Assuming approximately plane waves of ultrasound, the instantaneous intensity i in an ultrasonic field is given by:

$$i = \frac{p^2}{\rho c}$$

where p is the instantaneous excess acoustic pressue, ρ is the density of the medium and c is the speed of sound in the medium. If p is measured by a hydrophone of sensitivity k V/Pascal, then i is given by:

$$i = \frac{v^2}{k^2 \rho c}$$

22

where v is the instantaneous hydrophone voltage.
The temporal average intensity is given by

$$I_{TA} = \frac{1}{k^2\rho c} \frac{1}{(t_2-t_1)} \int_{t_1}^{t_2} v^2(t)dt \qquad (1)$$

where v(t) is the voltage waveform produced by the hydrophone and (t_2-t_1) is the pulse repetition period or the scan repetition period for real time systems.

(b)   Calculation of the temporal average intensity

(i)   Assumption of sinusoidal waveform
Equation (1) may be evaluated approximately by assuming that each half cycle of an ultrasonic pulse is a half cycle of a sine wave.
For a continuous sine wave:

$$I_{TA} = \frac{V^2}{2k^2\rho c} \qquad (2)$$

where V is the peak hydrophone voltage.
For a pulsed waveform, I_{TA} is given approximately by:

$$I_{TA} = \frac{1}{2k^2\rho c} \frac{T/2}{(t_2-t_1)} \sum_{i=1}^{N} V_i^2 \qquad (3)$$

where T/2 is the average duration of a half cycle of the pulse waveform, (t_2-t_1) is the pulse repetition period or the scan repetition period, V_i is the peak hydrophone voltage in the i th half cycle of the waveform and N is the number of half cycles in the pulse for static scanning systems or the number of half cycles in all the pulses received by the hydrophone during a complete scan in the case of real time systems.
Relatively accurate measurements of temporal average intensity can be obtained using this approximation for CW (using equation 2) and pulsed Doppler systems (equation 3) where the transmitted pulses are long and of low temporal peak intensity so that waveform distortion due to non-linear propagation in the water bath does not occur[4]. For single element imaging systems e.g. B-scanners, this measurement method is easy to implement as there is only one ultrasonic pulse per p.r.f. cycle to make measurements on. However, waveform distortion may give rise to inaccuracies in estimating V_i.

(ii)   Integration by computer graphics methods
Integration of individual ultrasonic pulse waveforms may be performed using computer graphics equipment such as a graphics tablet. A stable display of the hydrophone signal from each pulse to be integrated is produced on an oscilloscope screen. The display is then photographed and the resulting photographic image digitised by tracing out the pulse shape using a graphics tablet or other graphics digitising device. Equation (1) can then be evaluated for each digitised waveform by the associated computer. The pulses may be photographed on site and the photographs taken to the computer for analysis.
The computer graphics method of integration is able to allow for deviations from sinusoidal waveforms commonly encountered in pulse-echo imaging systems

but is usually not suitable for pulsed Doppler devices due to the difficulty of displaying and digitising pulses containing a large number of cycles.

(iii)   Real time systems
In the case of real time scanning systems such as linear arrays, the hydrophone is positioned at the point in the ultrasonic field where I_{TA} is to be measured. As the ultrasonic beam is swept past the hydrophone, a series of pulses is received from consecutive transmissions. The amplitudes of the pulses vary according to the position of the beam with respect to the position of the hydrophone, normally reaching a maximum when the beam axis intersects the hydrophone. Where interlacing techniques are used, the received pulse sequence may be different on alternate scans of the array and a relatively complex sequence may be received from arrays which use multiple zone focussing on transmit.

To make temporal average intensity measurements on such real time systems by analysis of individual pulses, it is necessary to have access to scan trigger signals inside the machine and to have a thorough understanding of the pulse transmission sequence so that each pulse in a complete scan sequence can be examined in turn using an oscilloscope with a delayed trigger facility. It is then necessary to make measurements on this large number of pulses for each machine/ transducer combination. Such techniques become impracticable for field measurements.

In the field it may only be possible to make approximate measurements of temporal average intensity on real time scanners by analysing only the largest pulse in the sequence. The contributions to the temporal average intensity from the other pulses in the sequence may then be estimated by assuming that the pulse shape is constant so that the contribution of each pulse is directly proportional to the square of its peak voltage. Only the relative amplitudes of all the other pulses in the sequence need then be measured.

In the case of mechanical sector scanners, it may be impossible to make temporal average intensity measurements in the scanning mode by integration of individual pulses as the positions of the transmitted beams usually vary from one scan to the next.

In short, reliable measurements of spatial peak, temporal average intensity can be difficult and time consuming to make on real time systems in the field by methods involving individual pulse analysis; an alternative method is desirable.

(iv)   Measurement of temporal average intensity with an r.f. power meter
The method of choice used by the author for measurements of I_{SPTA} employs an r.f. power meter. This power meter is a portable instrument and is used with a thermocouple sensor. The sensor contains a semiconductor Seebeck device which presents an input impendance of 50 Ω at the input terminal. The time averaged power into the 50 Ω is measured for any signal waveform applied to the input by measuring the average Seebeck potential produced.

The thermocouple sensor responds to signals in the frequency range 30 kHz to 4.2 GHz and can measure power in the range 1 μW to 100 mW. Because the sensor employs a thermal technique for power measurement, it works equally well for pulsed or continuous wave signals.

The r.f. power measurement system is illustrated in *figure 3.3*. The calibrated hydrophone is connected to the portable oscilloscope via a preamplifier. The oscilloscope contains an attenuator (the voltage range control) and a 60 MHz bandwidth amplifier. It has been modified to include an additional wideband

24

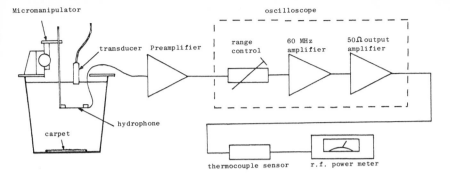

Figure 3.3   The r.f. power meter system used for measurement of I_{SPTA}.

amplifier stage after the 60 MHz amplifier which can give peak output voltages up to 3 V into a 50 Ω load. This 50 Ω output is connected to the power sensor. Using this arrangement, ultrasonic pulse waveforms displayed on the oscilloscope screen are given enough average power to be measured by the thermocouple sensor.

Equation (1) may be rewritten:

$$I_{TA} = \frac{R}{k^2 \rho c \, G^2(f)} \frac{G^2(f)}{R\,(t_2-t_1)} \int_{t_1}^{t_2} v^2\,(t)dt$$

where R is the input impedance of the thermocouple sensor (50Ω) and G(f) is the voltage gain of the preamplifier, oscilloscope range control, 60 MHz amplifier and 50Ω output amplifier chain.

The power P measured by the r.f. power meter is given by:

$$P = \frac{G^2(f)}{R\,(t_2-t_1)} \int_{t_1} v^2\,(t)dt$$

$$\text{Hence} \quad I_{TA} = \frac{R}{k^2 \rho c \, G^2(f)} \times P$$

The power gain $G^2(f)$ of the system has been measured using a continuous sine wave signal from a signal generator at frequencies in the range 1–10 MHz.

The temporal average intensity at the hydrophone may be calculated from the simplified equation:

$$I_{TA} = K(f) \times S^2 \times P \text{ mW cm}^{-2}$$

where K(f) is a factor which includes G(f), k, ρ, c and R. S is the voltage range setting of the oscilloscope (in volts/division) and P is the power meter measurement (in watts).

To check that the power meter system was able to make accurate measurements of temporal average intensity, the temporal average intensity at the spatial peak was measured for a series of B-scan transducers. In each case, after location of the spatial peak, the power meter reading was taken and the ultrasonic pulse was photographed from the oscilloscope screen with a polaroid camera. Each waveform was digitised from the photograph six times using an Apple microcomputer and graphics tablet. The mean value of I_{SPTA} calculated by the computer graphics method was compared with the value calculated from the power meter reading.

Table 3.1 Comparison of r.f. power meter and computer graphics methods of measurement of I_{SPTA} from B-scan transducers.

Frequency (MHz)	Diameter (mm)	Power meter measurement (mW cm^{-2})	Computer graphics measurement (mW cm^{-2})	
			mean	standard deviation
1.5	19	21.0	21.0	0.2
2.25	13	19.8	20.8	1.8
2.25	19	22.7	19.7	2.2
2.5	19	29.2	31.0	1.3
3.5	13	32.0	35.8	2.2
7.5	6	7.9	7.5	0.8

The results are shown in *table 3.1*. The power meter measurement is in each case within two standard deviations of the mean computer graphics measurement showing that the power meter measurement method does not give rise to any serious errors.

The r.f. power meter enables temporal average intensity measurements to be made rapidly and conveniently on all types of diagnostic ultrasound systems without internal triggering signals or detailed knowledge of the system operation.

(c) Location of the spatial peak of the temporal average intensity
The point of spatial peak temporal average intensity in the ultrasonic field is approached from the far field of the transducer (or from beyond the focus) to avoid confusion with near field maxima. The hydrophone is moved towards the transducer while making slight movements along the horizontal axes of the micromanipulator to verify that the hydrophone is on the beam axis. The signal is maximised iteratively along the three axes until the true point of spatial peak intensity is identified.

For non-auto scanning systems, the position of the spatial peak, temporal average intensity will normally correspond to the point where the hydrophone signal amplitude reaches a maximum. This may not be the case for real time systems however, where overlapping of consecutive beam positions can give rise to a larger temporal average intensity at some other depth. This effect leads to further uncertainty in calculations of I_{SPTA} by the methods of individual pulse integration. Using the power meter approach the temporal average intensity is measured at each point in the field making it possible to find the true point of spatial peak, temporal average intensity.

26

3.3.3 Spatial peak pulse average intensity

Spatial peak pulse average intensity (I_{SPPA}) is the intensity integral of the largest pulse in the ultrasonic field divided by the pulse duration. The AIUM/NEMA standard defines the pulse duration as 1.25 times the time interval between the points on the pulse waveform at which the pulse intensity integral is 0.1 and 0.9 of the total pulse intensity integral.

I_{SPPA} by this definition is most conveniently measured in the field by photographing the largest pulse and making the calculations back at base using a computer graphics digitiser with appropriate software.

Carson et al[5] have used an alternative definition to measure pulse average intensities. This is the average pulse intensity between the times t_1 and t_2 on the voltage waveform where t_1 and t_2 correspond to the times of zero crossing just prior to and just after the first and last times in the waveform at which $v(t)$ exceeds $0.25\ v(t)_{max}$. I_{SPPA} by this definition may be estimated in the field directly from the oscilloscope display using the half sine wave approximation (equation 3) if there is no significant waveform distortion.

3.3.4 Spatial average temporal average intensity

The spatial average temporal average intensity should be measured in the plane of the spatial peak temporal average intensity by averaging the temporal average intensity over the cross sectional area of the beam contained within the 6 dB contour, i.e. that part of the beam in which the temporal average intensity is greater than 25 per cent of I_{SPTA}[1]. This measurement requires the plotting of several beam profiles, a time consuming procedure using a manually operated hydrophone positioning device. An alternative acceptable definition for I_{SATA}[1] is:

$$I_{SATA} = \frac{W}{A_6}$$

where W is the total ultrasonic power (measured with the radiation force balance) and A_6 is the 6 dB area of the beam. For circular transducers, A_6 can be estimated from the 6 dB beam diameter in the plane of I_{SPTA} using the micromanipulator scale. A_6 for a linear array can be estimated from the 6 dB beam width and scan length.

I_{SATA} measurements are often quoted which have been made by dividing the total radiated power by the labelled active area of the transducer or array. This is a very simple measurement to make but does not fulfill the AIUM/NEMA definition as it does not yield the maximum value of I_{SATA} for any plane through the beam.

3.4 Summary of measurement procedure

For each machine/transducer combination, the total ultrasonic power is measured with all machine controls (e.g. transmitter power, p.r.f., scan angle) set to give the maximum possible reading. The transducer is then mounted over the water bath containing the hydrophone and the position of I_{SPTA} located using the micromanipulator and the r.f. power meter. The power meter reading is recorded and the 6 dB beam width measured using the micromanipulator scale for calculation of I_{SATA}. The largest pulse is then located and photographed for subsequent calculation of I_{SPPA}.

Acknowledgement

I am indebted to Mr P J Saunders for his modifications to the radiation force balance and for the computer software used to digitise and analyse the ultrasonic pulse waveforms. I would also like to thank Dr T A Whittingham for his helpful discussions.

References

1 AIUM/NEMA Standards Publication No UL1–1981 Safety standard for diagnostic Ultrasound Equipment *Journal of Ultrasound in Medicine* 2 S1–S49
2 FARMERY M J and WHITTINGHAM T A 1978 Portable radiation-force balance for use with diagnostic ultrasonic equipment *Ultrasound in Medicine and Biology* 3 373–379
3 CORNHILL C V 1982 Improvement of portable radiation force balance design *Ultrasonics* 20 282–284
4 STARRITT H C, DUCK F A and HUMPHREY V F 1983 Non-linear distortion of ultrasonic pulse shapes. HPA meeting on Physics in Medical Ultrasound, Durham, July 1983
5 CARSON P L, FISCHELLA P A and OUGHTON T V 1978 Ultrasonic power and intensities produced by diagnostic ultrasound equipment *Ultrasound in Medicine and Biology* 3 341–350

Appendix

Details of portable equipment

1. Portable radiation force balance
This balance is as described by Farmery and Whittingham[2] but modified by Mr P J Saunders so that it could be filled with distilled water rather than paraffin oil. The balance could then be used at ultrasonic frequencies up to 10 MHz without frequency related corrections. The modifications included the provision of extra electrical insulation and increased mechanical and electrical damping to offset the low viscosity of water.

2. Calibrated PVDF bilaminar hydrophone
The hydrophone (type Y–33–7611, 1 mm diameter active element) was supplied by Marconi Research Centre, West Hanningfield Road, Gt. Baddow, Chelmsford, Essex and calibrated by the National Physical Laboratory.

3. Hydrophone preamplifier
This device was supplied by Mr J P Weight of 'Festina', Luxford Road, Crowborough, East Sussex. The specification of the device included 6 pF input capacitance, 10 MΩ input resistance, 60 MHz bandwidth, 50 Ω output impedance and 10 dB gain (with a 1 kΩ load at the output).

4. Bucket, mounting plate and micromanipulator
The micromanipulator was supplied by Prior Scientific Instruments, London Road, Bishop's Stortford, Herts. A mounting plate to hold the micromanipulator over the plastic bucket was built in the Medical Physics mechanical workshop.

5. The oscilloscope (Tektronix type 2215)

This was modified to include graticule illumination and power supply for the hydrophone preamplifier. The 50 Ω output amplifier was based on the LH0032 operational amplifier and was capable of providing a peak voltage of 3 volts into a 50 Ω load at frequencies in the range of 100 kHz to 10 MHz (further details are available from the author).

6. Camera

A Shackman type 7000 polaroid camera was used to photograph the oscilloscope display.

7. R.F. Power meter

The r.f. power meter is type 6950 and the sensor type 6912 from Marconi Instruments Ltd, St Albans, Herts. The sensor can measure power in the range 1 μW to 100 mW (peak power 15 W for 2 μs) over a frequency range 30 kHz to 4.2 GHz. The response time of the power meter and sensor is continuously variable between 30 ms and 15 s using a rear panel control.

CHAPTER 4

A New Primary Standard for Hydrophone Calibration

D R Bacon, L E Drain*, B C Moss* and R A Smith
National Physical Laboratory, Teddington, Middlesex, and
(*) *Atomic Energy Research Establishment, Harwell, Oxfordshire*

4.1 Introduction

The requirement for determining absolutely the acoustic levels in the fields from medical ultrasonic equipment is commonly met by the use of miniature hydrophones. To provide absolute measurements, these hydrophones must be calibrated, and thus the primary calibration of hydrophones is of crucial importance.

A new standard technique for determining the free-field sensitivity of hydrophones has been developed at the National Physical Laboratory (NPL) under a co-operative project with AERE Harwell, which was partly funded by the Commission of the European Communities (Community Bureau of Reference, BCR). The method relies on the determination of the particle displacement in an ultrasonic field using a Michelson interferometer[1-3]. The acoustic pressure at a particular point in the field is derived from the displacement and a knowledge of the acoustic impedance of the propagating medium, and the hydrophone is then calibrated by placing it at the same point in the field and determining its output voltage.

The interferometer was originally developed at AERE Harwell[2] and has recently been improved to meet the requirements of the hydrophone calibration method. The most significant improvements were the extension of the frequency response and the reduction of the noise level. The first of these characteristics determines the absolute accuracy of the method, whilst the noise level determines the upper frequency limit of calibration.

At NPL, the interferometer has been incorporated into a calibration system and its performance has been assessed. Sources of systematic uncertainty that would influence the calibration result have been studied and, where possible, corrected for or eliminated. At present, calibrations have been performed up to a frequency of 15 MHz where the estimated overall uncertainty, which is predominantly systematic in origin, is ± 6.3 per cent.

4.2 Method

A schematic diagram of the system is shown in *figure 4.1*. The ultrasonic wave propagating in water is incident on a thin plastic pellicle supported in the beam, which follows the motion of the water particles. This pellicle is coated with an optically reflecting film of gold and its motion is detected by the signal beam of the interferometer which is focussed at the rear surface of the pellicle. Unfortunately, environmental vibration causes the pellicle to move, introducing changes of optical phase in the signal beam and generating spurious signals in the output of the interferometer. This problem is overcome by using a feedback system which

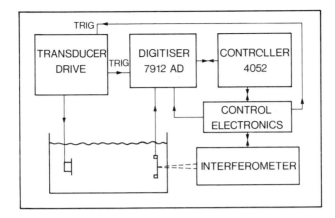

Figure 4.1   Block diagram of the system.

compensates for the phase changes due to vibration by introducing equal phase changes into the reference beam.

The compensation is achieved using an electro-optic Pockels cell to introduce a small frequency shift for the light in the reference beam. The compensation circuit does not respond to the high frequency ultrasonic signal, which is detected at the output. The interferometer is operated in such a way that, for small ultrasonic amplitudes (5 nm or less), the output signal amplitude, V_i, is directly proportional to the displacement. To determine the displacement absolutely it is necessary to know the reference voltage, V_o, which is the signal amplitude for a displacement corresponding to one or more fringes. The displacement amplitude of the ultrasonic wave, a, is given by

$$a \simeq \frac{V_i}{V_o} \frac{\lambda}{4\pi n^*} \tag{1}$$

where λ is the optical wavelength (in vacuum), and n^* is the effective refractive index of water. This approximate relationship is valid if $V_i \ll V_o$. The value of V_o depends on the amount of light reflected by the pellicle, and as this can vary due to the effect of environmental vibration it is desirable to measure V_i and V_o at the same instant. In practice, V_o can only be measured when the feedback circuit is switched off and thus V_o is actually determined 7 ms before and after the ultrasound is detected. To achieve this, the feedback circuit is automatically switched under computer control, and a sampling voltmeter used to determine V_o at the appropriate instant.

Having determined the displacement, the acoustic pressure can be calculated under the assumption of plane progressive wave propagation. If the pellicle is replaced by a hydrophone, with its active element at the point of intersection of the interferometer beam with the pellicle, then the sensitivity, M, can be determined using the equation

$$M \simeq \frac{V_h V_o}{V_i} \frac{2n^*}{f\rho c\lambda} \tag{2}$$

where V_h is the output voltage from the hydrophone, f is the ultrasonic frequency, ρ is the density of water and c is the sound velocity in water.

4.3 System performance

The accuracy of the calibration method is critically dependent on certain system parameters. The first parameter is the frequency response of the interferometer. This is important because the calculated sensitivity depends on the ratio V_o/V_i (equation 2) and V_o is determined at a frequency of approximately 2 kHz whilst V_i is measured in the megahertz frequency range. Various methods have been used to determine the frequency response, but it remains the least well-known characteristic of the system, giving rise to an uncertainty of $\pm$ 1 per cent at 0.5 MHz rising to $\pm$ 4.5 per cent at 15 MHz.

The hydrophone sensitivity is also determined by the ratio V_h/V_i (equation 2), and this depends on the linearity of the device used to measure the signals. By careful control of the measurement conditions it is estimated that this ratio can be determined with an accuracy of $\pm$ 0.1 per cent. Given that the ratio V_h/V_i and the frequency response are known, the sensitivity depends on the absolute accuracy of the measurement of V_o which is typically $\pm$ 0.25 per cent.

Other performance characteristics that affect the calibration accuracy are the reproducibility of the measurements and the noise level. The noise level is very important because, at the highest calibration frequencies, the displacement amplitude that can be obtained is very low (0.3 nm). Using narrowband detection with a 1 MHz bandwidth the noise level is 0.013 nm, giving a signal-to-noise ratio of at least 20. The reproducibility of the measurements depends on the experimental procedure, but in the present system, where approximately 1000 samples of V_i and 250 samples of V_h are taken, the standard deviation in the results is approximately 1 per cent.

4.4 Systematic effects

In the simplified explanation of the method given above, a number of assumptions were made, such as the assumption of plane wave propagation. These have been studied both experimentally and theoretically so that the measurement conditions can be arranged to minimise the influence of any systematic effects on the calibration results. Where necessary, the results of these studies have been applied to correct for any residual systematic effects.

The largest influence on the method is the acousto-optic interaction, which arises because the refractive index of water changes with pressure. The signal beam from the interferometer passes through the acoustic wave that has been transmitted by the pellicle, and consequently an interaction takes place. For a plane acoustic wave travelling in a direction parallel to the optical beam the effect can be accounted for simply[1] and is conveniently expressed by the use of an effective refractive index, n^* (which is 1.01 for water), instead of the true index. In a diffractive field there is a second type of contribution due to the acousto-optic interaction, but it can be shown that this effect is 0.1 per cent or less in magnitude, provided that the distance between the pellicle and radiating transducer is greater than ten transducer diameters.

A second factor that must be taken into account is the acoustical transmission coefficient of the pellicle. This, along with the reflection coefficient, has been determined experimentally at a range of frequencies and for pellicles of different thicknesses. By fitting a theoretical curve to these data, it is possible to predict the transmission of the pellicle at a particular frequency with an accuracy which is greater than that of the individual experimental result at the same frequency point.

The assumption of plane wave propagation is significant because it affects the accuracy of the method in several different ways: through the conversion from displacement to acoustic pressure, through the transmission properties of the pellicle and through the spatial averaging properties of the hydrophone. All of these effects have a similar dependence on the distance, r, between the pellicle and the transducer, being proportional to $b^2/(r^2 + b^2)$ provided r is sufficiently large, where b is the effective radius of the transducer.

The effect of diffraction on the relationship between particle displacement and pressure was included in the calculations of the acousto-optic interaction and the resulting uncertainty is $\pm$ 0.02 per cent or less for the calibration conditions employed. The spatial averaging effect arises because the interferometer detects the field at the focus of the signal beam, which is approximately 0.1 mm in diameter, whereas the hydrophone detects the acoustic pressure averaged over its active area, which is typically 1 mm in diameter. This effect is greatest at the highest calibration frequencies, because smaller propagation distances are used (in order to obtain higher signal levels) and because the effect depends on the ratio of the active element diameter to the acoustic wavelength. At 15 MHz the size of the correction is approximately 1 per cent, with an uncertainty of $\pm$ 0.4 per cent.

The acoustical transmission properties of a pellicle in a diffractive field are, in general, different from those in a plane wave. This is because the acoustic amplitude and phase vary across the membrane surface and it is therefore possible to excite plate waves. In general there can be a focussing effect, whereby the amplitude on the axis is greater when the pellicle is present than when it is absent. A theoretical study of this effect has shown that, for the pellicles and propagation distances used in calibration, the uncertainty introduced into the result is less than $\pm$ 0.1 per cent.

4.5   Results

A hydrophone has been calibrated using the interferometer at frequencies of 0.5, 1, 2, 3, 5, 7, 10 and 15 MHz. The overall uncertainty is obtained by adding the systematic components and then combining the sum in quadrature with the random uncertainty (95 per cent confidence level). The estimated overall uncertainty is $\pm$ 2.1 per cent at 0.5 MHz, $\pm$ 3.5 per cent at 10 MHz and $\pm$ 6.3 per cent at 15 MHz, representing an improvement in accuracy of a factor of 2.5 or more over the methods previously implemented at NPL. The results are in agreement with those of two other independent methods, reciprocity and planar scanning[4].

A comparison was also made between the frequency response of the hydrophone as determined by the interferometer, and as predicted by a previously developed theoretical model[5], and the results are presented in *figure 4.2*. Within the uncertainties of the calibration method, agreement is shown at all frequencies.

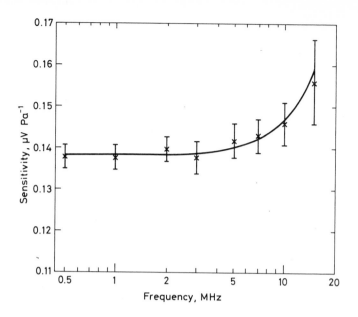

Figure 4.2 The sensitivity of a hydrophone as a function of frequency, obtained using the interferometric method. The error bars correspond to the estimated overall uncertainties. The continuous curve represents the predicted sensitivity, based on a theoretical model of the frequency response[5].

4.6 Conclusion

A primary hydrophone calibration method, based on laser interferometry, has been developed offering uncertainties of between 2.1 and 6.3 per cent in the frequency range 0.5 to 15 MHz. The method has been validated by a careful study of systematic effects and by intercomparison with alternative techniques. A reference hydrophone has been calibrated, and this now forms the basis of the calibration service offered to customers by the NPL.

There is still a requirement for further work on the method, particularly to redetermine the frequency response of the interferometer and to reduce the time taken for a calibration. As ultrasonic equipment is developed to operate at higher frequencies (such as the prototype scanner recently used to examine skin at 25 MHz[6]), there will be increasing requirements for measurements at frequencies above 15 MHz. It may thus become necessary to extend the frequency range of the hydrophone calibration method, and to do this it would be necessary to decrease the noise level from the interferometer by using a higher powered laser. Other possible developments include the use of the interferometer to measure ultrasonic fields directly, taking advantage of its high spatial resolution (0.1 mm), and the provision of calibrations at frequencies below 0.5 MHz, for applications such as surgery and dentistry.

Acknowledgements

The interferometer was developed and supplied by the Atomic Energy Research Establishment, Harwell, Didcot, Oxon OX11 0RA. The project was partly supported by a contract placed by the Commission of the European Communities, Bureau Communitaire de Reference.

References

1 MEZRICH R S, ETZOLD K F and VILKOMERSON D H R 1974 System for visualising and measuring ultrasonic wavefronts *RCA Review* **35** 483–519
2 SPEAKE J H 1978 An absolute method of calibrating ultrasonic transducers using laser interferometry *Proc Conference on The Evaluation and Calibration of Ultrasonic Transducers* 106–114 (IPC Science and Technology Press, Guildford, UK)
3 REIBOLD R and MOLKENSTRUCK W 1981 Laser interferometric measurement and computerised evaluation of ultrasonic displacements *Acustica* **49** 205–211
4 PRESTON R C, LIVETT A J and BACON D R 1984 Absolute calibration of hydrophones in the frequency range 0.5 MHz to 15 MHz *Proc Inst Acoust* **6** (Pt 5), 60–67
5 BACON D R 1982 Characteristics of a pvdf membrane hydrophone for use in the range 1–100 MHz *IEEE Trans Son Ultrason* **SU–29** 18–25
6 DINES K A, *et al* 1984 High frequency ultrasonic imaging of skin: experimental results *Ultrasonic Imaging* **6** 408–434

CHAPTER 5

IPSM Survey of Manufacturers Data of Diagnostic Ultrasound Equipment

D McHugh
Regional Department of Physics and Bioengineering, Christie Hospital,
Wilmslow Road, Manchester M20 9BX

5.1 Background

During the last year or so, there has been increasing concern among the general public about the safety of diagnostic ultrasound, particularly in the field of obstetrics. For several years the scientific community has urged caution over the use of ultrasound, because the basic interaction mechanisms of this form of energy with tissue are not fully understood. Against this background, several international bodies such as the World Health Organisation, the European Federation of Ultrasound in Medicine and Biology, as well as national groups of professionally concerned people such as the Royal College of Obstetricians and Gynaecologists [1] and the British Institute of Radiology have reviewed much of the experimental work published in this area. Government departments in the USA have also published information and guidelines on the biological effects of ultrasound [2,3]. Most of these groups have reached the same conclusion, and expressed the opinion that, where the ultrasound examination is of direct benefit to the patient, and the lowest practicable power is used, then the examination should be carried out. They have usually urged that further research should be carried out on the biological effects of ultrasound.

In 1976 the American Institute of Ultrasound in Medicine (AIUM) issued a statement on effects of ultrasound on tissue, that many people over the years have taken to be their licence to use ultrasound.

Statement on mammalian in-vivo ultrasonic biological effects. August 1976,
Revised October 1978, Reaffirmed October 1982

"In the low megahertz frequency range there have been (as of this date) no independently confirmed significant biological effects in mammalian tissues exposed to intensities* below 100 mW cm^{-2}. Furthermore, for ultrasonic exposure times** less than 500 seconds and greater than one second, such effects have not been demonstrated even at higher intensities, when the product of intensity* and exposure time** is less than 50 joules cm^{-2}."

Since this statement was issued in 1976, there has been a shift in attitude away from the idea that if the output is less than 100 mW cm^{-2} there is no need to worry, towards giving active consideration to the output of the machine, and operating it at the minimum power consistent with obtaining satisfactory information. Purchasers of ultrasound equipment are encouraged to ask for the output data and take this into account when purchasing new equipment.

* Spatial peak temporal average as measured in a free field in water.
** Total time: this includes off time as well as on time for a repeated pulse regime.

In 1981 the National Electrical Manufacturers Association (NEMA) together with the AIUM published a joint document entitled 'Safety Standard for Diagnostic Ultrasound Equipment'[4]. The purpose of this document was to lay down definitions of ultrasound parameters, primarily relating to acoustic output levels, specifying test methods where appropriate, as well as reviewing current information on biological effects. The stated object was to ensure that sufficient information on the characteristics of the equipment are properly determined to allow medical personnel to make informed judgements regarding the use of equipment on patients. It is not a mandatory standard, and lays down no maximum output levels. It is intended to be used as a guide, both by manufacturers and users and to introduce consistency in determining output parameters.

In the early 1980's the AIUM introduced a scheme to encourage manufacturers to make available acoustic output data. This involved supplying the AIUM with output data that could be made available to the public. Providing the AIUM approved the data they would award a commendation to the manufacturer for the specified machine and probes. The commendation was for making the data available and not specifically approving the machine as safe to use. In the rules attached to the award there is no mention of the criteria used to determine the award, although some companies that have applied have been turned down. The award lasts for one year and can be renewed following resubmission of data. While this scheme has limited value in controlling power output, it is the first real attempt to make data available to the user and it is gaining increasing acceptance. The 1985 AIUM awards booklet[5] lists 92 probes from 8 manufacturers and contains over 700 power and intensity values.

5.2 The IPSM Survey

In late 1984 the IPSM Ultrasound Topic Group decided to ask the manufacturers of diagnostic ultrasound equipment for the output data of the machines that they marketed in this country. If the encouragement given to users by advisory bodies over the last few years had had any effect this should have been a simple exercise; in fact it proved to be protracted and difficult.

The Ultrasound Topic Group devised a form (*figure 5.1*) which requested acoustic power output information of the kind now required by the Food and Drug Administration in the USA. All manufacturers of ultrasound equipment

Table 5.1 Companies included in the survey.

Acuson	I.G.E.	SIEL
American Hospital Supply	Hewlett Packard	Siemens
Appleton	Honeywell	Sonicaid
Bruel & Kjaer	Kontron	Sonotron
Diagnostic Sonar	Kretz	Squibb Medical
Doptek	Medisonics	Toshiba
Dynamic Imaging	Parks	Technicare
Elscint	Picker	Vingmed
GL Ultrasound	Philips	

must submit data on the output of new equipment before they can begin marketing it in the USA. This is a mandatory requirement, however the data supplied is not made public. The Topic Group requested data on the basis that a range of values would be published but in such a way as not to identify individual machines or companies. The companies circulated are given in *table 5.1*. Some companies are subsidiaries of the manufacturer and some are agents. Some of the agents handle the machines of several different manufacturers.

ACOUSTIC OUTPUT LEVELS

Name of manufacturer:

Equipment brand name and model:

Model number of transducer:

Mode of operation (e.g. B-scan, Doppler etc.):

Type of scan if appropriate (e.g. sector, linear etc.):

Frequency of operation: MHz

Total ultrasonic power: mW

Spatial average temporal average intensity: $mW\ cm^{-2}$

Spatial peak temporal average intensity: $mW\ cm^{-2}$

Spatial peak temporal peak intensity: $mW\ cm^{-2}$

Spatial peak pulse average intensity: $mW\ cm^{-2}$

Please provide details below of the method used to determine the acoustic levels. This should include the type of measurements used (e.g. hydrophone (type etc.), radiation balance, etc.), the sensitivity and the total uncertainty in the measurements. If possible an estimate of the type-testing uncertainty (the difference expected between nominally identical machines) should also be supplied.

Figure 5.1 Enquiry form circulated to manufacturers.

5.3 Results of the survey

Replies were received from 14 companies (60 per cent), with data promised from a further 4 which never materialised.

Inevitably the information received was very variable. It ranged from detailed information of output and explanation of how these were carried out, (mostly from USA-based manufacturers), to a simple statement of 'it's well within the 100 mW cm^{-2} value!'. This machine was not included in the data reported.

To measure the output of a modern machine such as a combined linear/sector device with pulsed wave Doppler option is a time-consuming and expensive undertaking. The machine will have several probes, some of which may have variable transmit focus, and M–mode. Each probe in every mode must be measured. To fully characterise a probe from a pulsed Doppler unit where the gate length, gate depth and pulse repetition frequency (PRF) all interact with each other, demands careful experimental work.

A few of the firms supplied detailed descriptions of how the outputs were measured. In most cases power was measured using a radiation force balance with an absorber attached to a balance, though there were variations of this principle. Two firms indicated they had determined power from the spatial average temporal average (SATA) intensity measurement and beam area data. The intensity measurements were usually carried out using a PVDF hydrophone, either the larger membrane type with a small active area or the small cone shaped devices. Some measurements were made using a ceramic hydrophone. Calibration was seldom mentioned. In the instances where reference was made to calibration, the company either relied on the original hydrophone data or checked it against other standards traceable to a national standard.

Few errors were quoted in the figures that were supplied. The NEMA Standard (4: page S8) suggest the maximum errors at the 68 per cent (1σ) confidence level should be less than ± 25 per cent for spatial peak temporal peak (SPTA), ± 30 per cent for SATA and ± 35 per cent for spatial peak pulse average (SPPA). The labelling of power output should be within ± 20 per cent. The errors given ranged from an optimistic ± 10 per cent to a carefully calculated ± 39 per cent. Until more critical standards are laid down and complied with, for calibration and measurement techniques, it will still be difficult to make a true assessment of the output data of different machines.

In order to illustrate the type of information supplied and the difficulties involved in carrying out these measurements an outline of the method used by one manufacturer will be given.

5.3.1 Example of output data measurement

The equipment operates over a range of PRFs depending on the machine settings. To simplify measurements all readings for all parameters are made at one PRF and corrected for the maximum possible output value. This assumes that power and temporal average intensities are proportional to PRF.

The machine was a single element mechanical sector scanner and all measurements were made with the crystal stationary and aligned along the axis of the probe. The intensity values were corrected for real-time scanning.

The power was measured, using the radiation force balance principle, with an acoustic absorber connected to a sensitive (100 μg) electrobalance. The force balance was calibrated using a quartz transducer whose output value was traceable to the NBS standard in the USA.

The probe was coupled to the window of the tank with gel and a series of 6 readings were made for each probe. The variation in these 6 values ranged from 2 per cent to 30 per cent depending on the probe under investigation. In each case the highest measured value was quoted for the power output of the probe.

Intensity measurements were made with a PVDF hydrophone using the makers calibration. The probe was coupled with gel to the side window of a plotting tank, and the hydrophone scanned through the beam to determine the position of the maximum intensity. The maximum signal was assessed by eye and the trace was photographed, copied, digitised by hand and the square of the voltage integral calculated for the duration of the pulse. The SPTA intensity is calculated using equation 1.

$$\frac{1}{k_f^2 \, (t_2 - t_1)} \int_{t_1}^{t_2} v^2 \, (t) dt \qquad (1)$$

where k_f is the intensity response factor of the hydrophone, t_1 and t_2 are the beginning and end of the pulse as defined in the NEMA standard, and v is the voltage measured by the hydrophone.

This value of SPTA is for a stationary transducer and will only apply to the M-mode. The real-time mode must be modified by the factor

$$\frac{\text{frame rate}}{\text{PRF}}$$

and an over-scan factor to take account of the fact that each point in the tissue will receive several pulses because of the finite beam width. In this case the factor was

Table 5.2 Range of output data supplied by manufacturers.

Machine	Power (mW)	I_{SATA} (mW cm^{-2})	I_{SPTA} (mW cm^{-2})	I_{SPTP} (W cm^{-2})	I_{SPPA} (W cm^{-2})
Linear array	0.063–55	0.045–11 (0.4–10)	0.02–48 (0.1–12)	4–830	0.4–310 (0.5–280)
Phased array	6.5–74	0.13–4	0.15–85	17–870	5–720
Mechanical sector	0.17–134	0.25–58 (2.7–60)	0.5–440 (45–200)	90–540	12–362 (25–100)
Static B-scanner	0.6–9	ND (0.4–20)	11–80 (10–100)	ND	24–109 (0.8–200)
Doppler CW obstetric monitors	17–24	4–14 (3–25)	7.2–27 (9–75)	14–75	—
Doppler CW vascular	3–57	41–73 (38–840)	85–215 (110–2500)	170–308	—
Doppler PW	18–64	50–560 (3–32)	40–940 (50–290)	20–137	7–69 (3–14)

estimated to be 3. In this way the SPTA was calculated for each probe for real-time B-mode scanning.

The SPPA was also calculated from the peak intensity integral and pulse duration. However in this case no attempt was made to measure any of the spatial average intensities.

One of the probes could not be operated in the stationary mode for technical reasons and the SPTA and SPPA were estimated from the power measurements and geometrical considerations.

As can be seen from this example there can be considerable deviation from the NEMA standards in practical output measurements. When such figures are quoted without supporting information it is impossible to judge their validity.

The range of the data received is presented in *table 5.2*, with the ranges given in the NEMA document shown in brackets.

The table shows an enormous range of values within one type of scanner. For example the linear array with the lowest power output quoted is a 5 MHz device while the one with the highest power output is a comparable machine with a 3.5 MHz probe, although there is a factor of almost 1,000 difference in their ouput. Over the whole range of imaging machines, the lowest outputs tend to be the general-purpose diagnostic devices and those at the higher end of the range the more specialised high frequency devices such as intra-operative probes, though several conventional cardiac scanners feature at this end of the range. The probe with the highest SPTA value is a 10 MHz mechanical sector scanner.

The number of replies relating to phased array, static B-scanners and Doppler machines are very small and may not be representative.

The data are presented in a more comprehensive form in *figures 5.2 to 5.7* which show the distribution of machines for each type of scanner and parameter.

Power
Figure 5.2 shows the power levels for each type of scanner. Each value recorded represents one probe. Linear array scanners have the lowest average power with most machines operating at less than 30 mW. Mechanical sector scanners show a greater spread but this reflects the greater number of specialist probes. All the static B-scanners have similar low outputs.

Spatial Average Temporal Average Intensity
Figure 5.3 shows the SATA levels and again the linear arrays have the lowest values. This is one of the more difficult measurements to make and was often not quoted. The highest value of 64 mW cm^{-2} is a 3.5 MHz mechanical sector for cardiac work with a corresponding SPTA intensity of 67 mW cm^{-2}.

Spatial Peak Temporal Average
The SPTA is the value referred to in the AIUM statement. Most of the imaging machines are below the 100 mW cm^{-2} value. The two quoted that are 380 and 440 mW cm^{-2} are very high frequency specialised mechanical scanners. The figures used to compile the chart do not include the values for real-time machines operating in the m-mode. In this case, the beam is stationary and frequently the PRF is increased to give better response to high speed reflectors. This can increase the SPTA value by a factor of 3 or more.

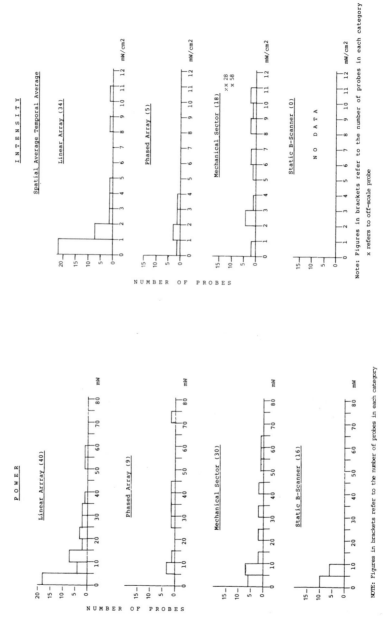

Figure 5.2 Histograms of power levels for each type of scanner. Each value recorded represents one probe.

Figure 5.3 Histograms of SATA levels of intensity.

42

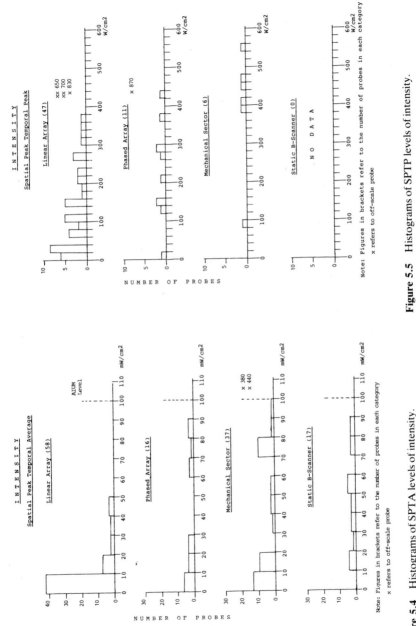

Figure 5.5 Histograms of SPTP levels of intensity.

Figure 5.4 Histograms of SPTA levels of intensity.

43

Spatial Peak Temporal Peak
The SPTP value is the highest recorded intensity as it represents the maximum total excursion (positive and negative) of the pressure at a point. There is usually a significant difference between the positive and negative half of the pressure cycle, which may have different biological significance. The highest recorded value is for a general purpose 5 MHz phased array probe, though several linear array devices come close behind.

Spatial Peak Pulse Average
Figure 5.6 shows the SPPA. This is a measure of the average energy in a pulse, and is considered to be one of the most useful parameters in assessing relative hazard. Again there was considerable variation among machines with similar performance, but some of the phased arrays were noticeably higher than other scanners.

Doppler-Continuous Wave
Power is little different from the imaging devices (*figure 5.7*), but as one would expect, the SATA of obstetric monitors is very low indicating a large beam area. The vascular machines are much higher with one exceeding 100 mW cm^{-2} for SPTA.

Doppler-Pulsed Wave
Power is a little higher than from continuous wave machines but the SATA is much higher because of smaller beam areas. The SPTA values are very high with one 10 times the 100 mW cm^{-2} level. This is a 3.5 MHz mechanical sector operating in the pulsed Doppler mode. It should be stressed that these are the worst case values, with maximum possible PRF.

5.4 General observations on the data and survey

1. The higher frequency probes tend to have lower power output, but the SATA intensity is similar for different frequencies because high frequency probes have smaller beam areas.

2. Usually the SPTA intensity is greater for higher frequency probes, because they are more strongly focussed.

3. Although the response to the survey was only 60 per cent after several reminders, this was thought to be because the information requested was not readily available, rather than any desire for commercial secrecy on the part of the companies. It appears that the information, when it is measured, is not widely distributed to the agents. It took some time for the agents in this country to extract information from the parent company in Japan or the USA. Often the form of the information was difficult to interpret as there was sometimes little detail on the methods used, or data was only partly translated from the original language. There were a few notable exceptions, particularly among those companies that had submitted data to the AIUM to obtain their manufacturers commendation. Even here however, it was usually only one or two models that were submitted and even then not all the transducers. One manufacturer published the information in the operators' manual and one in their sales brochure.

4. In most instances it took several months to get hold of the information, which indicated that very few users ask the sales-person for power output data.

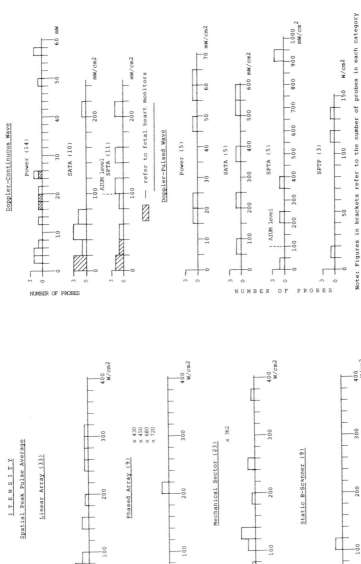

Figure 5.7 Histograms of power and intensity levels of Doppler CW and Doppler PW machines.

Figure 5.6 Histograms of SPPA levels of intensity.

45

Almost no sales people carry this data among their glossy brochures. Even detailed information on the range of transducers available is not always readily available.

5.5 Conclusions

This survey has shown that the range of acoustic output values has increased since the NEMA publication of 1981. There have been dramatic reductions in the output of some equipment, but there have also been some significant increases as well. These are most apparent for machines operating in the pulsed Doppler mode as well as for high frequency specialised probes.

The AIUM is to be encouraged in its endeavours to make output data more widely available. However there is a need for more well-defined methods of measuring parameters, and some way of persuading manufacturers to follow them. Only in this way can true comparisons be made of published data.

In recent years buyers have been encouraged to consider the relative acoustic outputs of machines with comparable performance, but judging from the difficulty encountered in obtaining this information very few people pursue the matter. There is, of course little point in asking for the information if one is not able to make any use of it, and the power output of one machine in isolation is of little use. The data is still in a rather complex form, and without any clear guidelines on the biological significance, a prospective purchaser can do little more than choose a machine that has outputs towards the lower end of the range. Bodies such as AIUM and individuals asking questions about output can raise everyone's awareness of output data, and thereby discourage manufacturers from increasing outputs. From a knowledge of the machines included in this survey the author concludes that the imaging performance of scanners bears no relation to their output. For example, it should be possible to purchase a reasonable linear array with an output of less than 10 mW and a SPPA of less than 20 W cm^{-2}, though the final patient exposure will still rely on the efficient use of the machine by the operator.

References

1 ROYAL COLLEGE OF OBSTETRICIANS AND GYNAECOLOGISTS 1984 *Report of the RCOG Working Party on Routine Ultrasound Examination in Pregnancy* (RCOG, 27 Sussex Place, Regents Park, London NW1 4RG)
2 BUREAU OF RADIOLOGICAL HEALTH 1982 *An Overview of Ultrasound: Theory, Measurement, Medical Applications, and Biological Effects* Report FDA 82–8190 (BRH, Rockville, Maryland 20857, USA)
3 NATIONAL COUNCIL OF RADIATION PROTECTION AND MEASUREMENTS 1983 *Biological Effects of Ultrasound: Mechanisms and Clinical Implications* Report 74 (NCRP Publications, 7910 Woodmont Avenue, Bethesda, Matyland 20814, USA)
4 NEMA/AIUM 1981 *Safety Standard for Diagnostic Ultrasound Equipment* AIUM/ NEMA III Standard Publication UL 1–1981 (NEMA 2101 L Street NW, Washington DC 20037, USA)
5 AMERICAN INSTITUTE OF ULTRASOUND IN MEDICINE 1985 *1985 Acoustical Data for Diagnostic Ultrasound Equipment* AIUM, 4405 East-West Highway, Suite 504, Bethesda, Maryland 20814, USA

CHAPTER 6

A Survey of the Output of Diagnostic Ultrasound Equipment

F A Duck, H C Starritt and A J Hawkins
Medical Physics Department, Royal United Hospital, Bath BA1 3NG

6.1 Introduction

Values of output acoustic parameters for diagnostic ultrasound units are only now beginning to become generally available. There have been two surveys which are commonly referred to, which have been quoted in most recent overviews of ultrasonic output values[1,2]. Both of these are somewhat dated. Hill's survey contains no data from focused transducers and Carson's, whilst more extensive and including focused fields, gives values from only two early linear arrays and one mechanical real-time scanner. Data for arrays are given in another publication[3] but many of the units surveyed were not strongly focused. In a recent publication[4] we have given more extensive and up-to-date figures for a wider range of scanners. We present here a summary of the values given in that paper, extended by some additional measurements on phased arrays and other linear arrays, and detailed values of measurements on pulsed Doppler and duplex systems. It should be noted at the outset that all values given in this paper are from individual units in clinical use, and cannot necessarily be used to charaterise all similar units from the same manufacturer.

6.2 Measurement details

The details of the measurement methods used are given elsewhere[4] but will be repeated in brief for completeness. The philosophy of the survey was to make adequately detailed measurements on as large a range of equipment in clinical use as possible. This placed constraints on the way in which the measurements were carried out and on the choice of measurement equipment. The majority of the scanners could not be moved from their clinical location, and thus the measurement equipment needed to be portable. Large automatic scanning tanks would not have been suitable. Furthermore, most of the scanners were in almost continual use leaving little time for detailed beam plotting. The measurements described below were designed so that an adequate characterisation of one beam could be completed within one morning or one afternoon.

Measurements were made using a calibrated polyvinylidene difluoride (PVDF) hydrophone to give information on the pressure waveform in water and on the variation of pressure in the beam. From these measurements values of pulse length, beam width, intensity and shock parameter were derived. Separately and independently measurements of total power were made whenever possible using an ultrasonic force balance, of a design similar to that described by Farmery and Whittingham[5]. These power measurements, and spatial-average intensities derived from them, provided confirmation of the correctness of values of intensity derived from the hydrophone measurements. It was not possible to make power measurements on linear arrays.

One of two alternative hydrophones was used to measure the pressure waveforms in water. The majority of measurements were made using a bilaminar screened PVDF membrane hydrophone 2×25 μm thick with a 1 mm diameter sensitive area (GEC–Marconi Electronics Ltd). The characteristics of this type of hydrophone, and its suitability for the measurement of pulsed ultrasonic fields have been described by Preston et al[6]. The second hydrophone used was a PVDF needle probe hydrophone, 0.6 mm diameter, 25 μm thick (Medicoteknisk Institute, Copenhagen). This hydrophone was used when higher spatial resolution was required, and in particular for beams whose half-amplitude beam-width was less than 1.5 mm. It was also used to confirm the pressure measurements made with the membrane hydrophone on a few machines, and also to provide an oscilloscope trigger for the array measurements.

The measurements were made in a small perspex tank (50×20 cm) with an acoustic absorber at the end, filled to an adequate depth immediately prior to the measurements with tap water. Gas bubbles tended to form under these conditions and it was necessary to continually clear them from the hydrophone and transducer using a brush. The transducer was held in a clamp on a retort stand and whenever possible it was immersed in the water, if necessary using greased plastic water proofing around the electrical connections. Some arrays were investigated by coupling the transducer through a thin plastic membrane window. All measurements were made with the acoustic axis horizontal. The hydrophone was mounted on a micromanipulator giving the ability to locate its position in three orthogonal directions to 0.1 mm. It was not possible to rotate either the transducer or the hydrophone in a controlled way. It was found possible however to align the hydrophone accurately with respect to the beam axis by iteratively adjusting the positions to maximise the hydrophone response at two axial locations. The hydrophone was connected directly to a Tektronix 465 oscilloscope, and overall peak voltages read directly. The NPL end-of-cable open circuit calibration figures were corrected for loading by the oscilloscope. Triggering was arranged in one of three ways. If the driving pulse was easily accessible it was used. Alternatively it was commonly found that a single wire aerial in the vicinity of the transducer gave a satisfactory trigger pulse. Triggering from arrays was not possible using either of these methods, and for arrays the two hydrophones were used together, one to provide an acoustically generated trigger, and the other for measurement.

In the majority of cases axial pressure variations were first measured, and followed by two beam profile measurements, one through the point of overall maximum pressure and a second as close to the transducer face as possible. Two orthogonal profiles were measured on arrays. The pulse waveform at the location of maximum pressure was recorded on polaroid film, and subsequently enlarged and digitised by hand in order to derive intensity and pulse length values. The pulse-average intensity and pulse length was estimated using the expressions given in the AIUM/NEMA standard[7] and more detail is given in chapter 8 of these Proceedings[8]. Pulse repetition rate and scan repetition rate were measured and together with pulse length used to derive values for temporal averaged intensities. Account was taken of the extent to which beam overlap occurred when estimating temporal average intensities for real-time systems while scanning. It should be emphasised that the derived values for intensity are not necessarily true spatial peak intensity values since it appears that the location of spatial peak pressure does not, in general, coincide with the location of spatial peak intensity. Experimental observations to support this assertion are given in chapter 8[8].

6.3 Results

Results from the survey are given in *tables 6.1* and *6.2*. *Table 6.1* summarises the results of all the measurements on imaging scanners including three B-scanners, four mechanical sector scanners, six linear array scanners and two phased array scanners. Details of most of the data from which this table was generated are to be found elesewhere[4]. Separate measurements were made if several transmit focus positions were available on linear arrays giving a total of 37 separate pulse-echo fields in all. The table summarises the results when equipment was at maximum power. As can be seen the range of frequencies was 2.0 to 7.1 MHz, and pulse lengths 0.12 to 1.23 μs. Direct measurements of power, made using the power balance, were used to derive values for spatial-average intensity at the transducer in all non-scanning conditions, I_{SATA} reaching a maximum of 370 W m^{-2} (10 W m^{-2} = 1 mW cm^{-2}). The highest peak pressure at the transducer of 1.30 MPa (approximately 13 atmospheres) was measured from a phased array. At the location of peak pressure, the highest positive pressure measured was 7.4 MPa, and the highest negative pressure–3.9 MPa. The spread of intensity values, pulse-averaged and temporal averaged, is shown in *figure 6.1* together with values

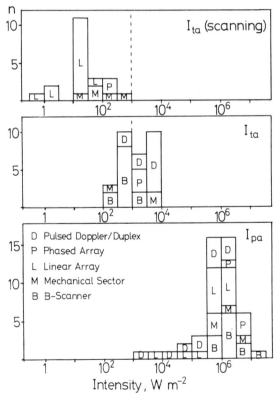

Figure 6.1 Histograms of all maximum intensity values obtained in the survey, separated by equipment type: Temporal average intensities while stationary and while scanning are shown separately, (I_{TA} and I_{TA} (scanning)). The dotted line is at 100 mW cm^{-2}. Pulse average intensities I_{PA} are shown at the bottom.

49

Table 6.1 Summary of maximum and minimum values for all measurements from pulse-echo equipment.

Parameter (units)	B-Scanner Transducers 3 Scanners 12 Transducers		Mechanical Sectors 4 Scanners 5 Scan-heads		Linear Arrays 6 Scanners 16 Arrays/Foci		Phased Arrays 2 Scanners 4 Arrays	
	Min	Max	Min	Max	Min	Max	Min	Max
Zero Cross. Freq. (MHz)	2.0	7.1	2.2	3.6	2.8	4.5	3.1	4.5
Pulse Length (μs)	0.12	0.60	0.40	0.84	0.33	1.23	0.17	0.35
Power (mW)	0.5	9.1	5.2	80	—	—	—	—
p+ at Transducer (MPa)	0.27	1.15	0.34	0.52	0.03	0.82	—	1.30
I_{SATA} at Transducer (W m^{-2})	10	78	53	370	—	—	—	—
At peak pressure:								
p+, (MPa)	2.1	6.5	2.1	7.4	0.1	3.9	4.0	7.4
p-, (MPa)	-0.9	-3.9	-0.9	-2.1	-0.1	-1.8	-2.3	-2.9
I_{PA} (W m^{-2})	3.6×10^5	1.1×10^7	3.3×10^5	3.2×10^6	3.6×10^3	1.6×10^6	2.0×10^6	5.4×10^6
I_{TA} (stopped) (W m^{-2})	1.9×10^2	1.8×10^3	2.4×10^2	6.8×10^3	0.7	32	152	204
I_{TA} (scanning) (W m^{-2})	—	—	2.2	370	0.1	3.2	—	—
σ_m	1.2	3.2	1.1	2.7	—	—	—	—

50

Table 6.2 Details of measurements from Duplex and pulsed Doppler units. + indicates that power control was available. Details of units A to J are given in *table 6.3*.

Code	Power Control	Zero Cross. Freq. (MHz)	prf (kHz)	Pulse Length (μs)	Power (mW)	$\hat{p}+$ (MPa)	$\hat{p}-$ (MPa)	Position of $\hat{p}+$ (mm)	I_{TA} (W m^{-2})	I_{PA} (W m^{-2})	σ_m
A (i)	+	3.0	4.8	0.87	46	3.85	−1.55	45	5.5×10^3	1.5×10^6	1.5
A (ii)	+	3.0	18.5	5.77	22	0.30	−0.26	45	3.0×10^3	2.8×10^4	0.2
B (i)		3.0	3.1	0.86	27	4.10	−1.50	53	3.3×10^3	1.1×10^6	2.5
B (ii)		3.0	18.7	10.00	5.6	0.12	−0.12	50	3.6×10^2	1.9×10^3	0.1
C (i)		4.4	7.9	0.44	—	3.35	−0.93	33	4.0×10^3	1.2×10^6	1.3
C (ii)		4.5	23.2	6.7	—	0.56	−0.33	44	5.7×10^3	3.7×10^4	0.4
D (i)		4.4	6.1	1.13	9.5	2.01	−1.25	30	4.6×10^3	6.8×10^5	0.9
D (ii)		4.4	15.0	10.6	6.0	0.29	−0.29	30	4.5×10^3	2.8×10^4	0.2
E		2.25	13.1	1.51	27	0.76	−0.58	35	3.1×10^3	1.5×10^5	0.3
F		3.5	13.1	1.17	14	0.94	−0.74	35	3.4×10^3	2.2×10^5	0.5
G	+	3.5	7.7	1.00	—	1.91	−0.74	75	2.6×10^3	3.3×10^5	—
H	+	5.0	7.7	0.74	—	2.09	−0.96	35	3.1×10^3	5.4×10^5	—
I		5.0	37	2.4	6.7	0.22	−0.22	15	1.5×10^3	1.7×10^4	—
J		10.0	46.5	1.3	—	0.10	−0.10	35	1.7×10^2	2.8×10^3	—

51

Table 6.3 Details of Duplex and Pulsed Doppler equipment investigated.

Code	Manufacturer	Scanner	Transducer	Operating Conditions
A (i) (ii)	A.T.L.	MK 600	Duplex	S.V. 1.5 mm; Max Depth 15 cm S.V. 9 mm; Max Depth 3 cm
B (i) (ii)	Diasonics	DRF 400	CMS D	S.V. 1 mm; prf 3.13 kHz S.V. 15.3 mm; prf 18.7 kHz
C (i) (ii)	Diasonics	DRF 400	SP/D 10	S.V. 0.6 mm; prf 7.8 kHz S.V. 10.2 mm; prf 15.6 kHz
D (i) (ii)	Technicare	Autosector	MOD 8107D	S.V. 1 mm; prf 3 kHz S.V. 8 mm; prf 7.5 kHz
E	Honeywell	UltraImager	Rt. Angle L Focus	
F	Honeywell	UltraImager	Rt. Angle S Focus	
G	Hewlett Packard	Imaging System	21205B M	Cursor 8 cm; Depth 12 cm
H	Hewlett Packard	Imaging System	21211A S	Cursor 8 cm; Depth 12 cm
I	Vingmed	Alfred	5 MHz	
J	Vingmed	Alfred	10 MHz	

for pulsed Doppler systems and are discussed further below. No values are given for temporal-peak intensity. The relationship $I = \hat{p}^2/\rho c$ has been widely used to calculate temporal-peak intensity from the measurement of the peak pressure $\hat{p}$ in the largest half cycle. However, considering the large measurement uncertainties for $\hat{p}$ resulting from the highly distorted wave patterns in the field together with the inadequate temporal and spatial response of the hydrophone, it was felt that it would be misleading to give values of peak intensity derived from these measurements. The extent to which finite-amplitude effects are important can be characterised using the non-linearity parameter σ. An expression developed by Bacon[9] for σ_m in a focused beam has been used and for nineteen out of 25 measurements where a calculation of σ_m was possible, $\sigma_m \geq 1.5$. Bacon gives an upper theoretical limit for σ_m of π, and for $\sigma_m \geq 1.5$ considerable finite amplitude distortion with amplitude loss of greater than 25 per cent from the fundamental has occurred.

Greater detail is given in *table 6.2* for pulsed Doppler fields from five duplex scanners and one peripheral vascular unit. The ten transducers and scanning heads investigated are listed in *table 6.3*. Output power was maximum and a note is made against those units where this could be reduced. Pulsed Doppler units can vary considerably in their pulsing characteristics and results from two extreme examples have been listed to allow some intercomparison between machines to be made. Broadly the conditions of smallest and largest sample volume (varying pulse length) and deepest and shallowest scan depth (varying prf) were used. They do not necessarily include settings giving absolute maximum temporal average intensity values, although it seems unlikely that the highest intensities are significantly higher than those given. The frequency range was 3.0 to 10.0 MHz. The pulse lengths ranged from 0.44 to 10.6 μs and the prf range was 3.1 to 46.5 kHz. Values of peak pressure and σ_m were generally slightly lower in extreme values than those obtained from pulse-echo units. Generally increases in pulse repetition rates were accompanied by a reduction in pressure and pulse average intensity resulting in little change in temporal-average intensity as the operating conditions varied.

A summary of all temporal-average and pulse-average intensities for pulse-echo and pulsed Doppler fields is shown in *figure 6.1*. Three separate histograms showing temporal average intensities in stationary and scanning modes, and pulse average intensity are presented. The complete span of intensities covers seven orders of magnitude. The lowest value of temporal average intensity whilst scanning for one linear array is less than 0.1 mW cm^{-2}; the highest value of 1.1 kW cm^{-2} pulse average intensity was found from one B-scan transducer. It is noticeable that 17 out of 30 measurements of temporal average intensity in a non-scanning mode (for instance B-scan, M-mode or pulsed Doppler) exceeded 100 mW cm^{-2} and that all three phased arrays and the majority of pulsed Doppler systems exceeded this threshold. The majority of temporal average intensities whilst scanning fell in the range 10 to 30 W m^{-2}, and 32 out of 47 measurements of pulse average intensity lie between 3×10^5 and 3×10^6 W m^{-2}.

6.4 Discussion

It has been found possible to carry out sensible dosimetry measurements for a survey of diagnostic ultrasound equipment using hydrophones and a power balance. A single set of measurements can be made at a clinical site (rather than in a laboratory) within half a day. While the power balance is specialised and is not

53

available commercially, facilities to make hydrophone measurements may be established by any centre following a relatively modest financial outlay. A suitable membrane hydrophone can be purchased, calibrated, for less than £1,000, and the remaining pieces of equipment, a micromanipulator, tank and oscilloscope with a 20 MHz bandwidth, are readily obtained. The ability to rotate the hydrophone and/or transducer in a controlled way would be a valuable addition. A second hydrophone is necessary if access to an electronic trigger from arrays is not possible.

Three particular aspects of the hydrophone deserve brief comment. The 1 mm diameter sensitive area was too large to allow correct measurement on the narrower focus beams and it is felt that a membrane hydrophone with a 0.5 mm sensitive area is in general required. We have indirect evidence that the spatial smoothing resulting from the use of too large a hydrophone has resulted in significant underestimates of peak pressure, particularly positive peak pressure, in some cases. Secondly the use of a bilaminar screened hydrophone has been found to be more convenient than the alternative of a coplanar screen hydrophone. A bilaminar hydrophone does not require the use of distilled water, is more reliable when used to generate a trigger signal, and the calibration does not depend upon the depth of immersion. Finally, the major problem concerning good quality measurements using a hydrophone has to do with hydrophone/cable resonance. The use of a broad band buffer amplifier at the hydrophone together with the use of thinner PVDF membranes in hydrophone construction will go a long way to alleviate this problem.

References

1 HILL C R 1971 Acoustic intensity measurements on ultrasonic diagnostic devices *Ultrasonographia Medica; 1st International Congress of Medical Ultrasonics, 2*, Eds Bock and Ossoinig, (Vienna Academy of Medicine, Vienna), pp 21–27
2 CARSON P L, FISCHELLA P R and OUGHTON T V 1978 Ultrasonic power and intensities produced by diagnostic ultrasound equipment *Ultrasound in Med & Biol* 3 341–350
3 DEPARTMENT of HEALTH and SOCIAL SECURITY 1979 Evaluation of real-time ultrasonic scanners; first report *Health Equipment Information* 81
4 DUCK F A, STARRITT H C, AINDOW J D, PERKINS M A and HAWKINS A J 1985 The output of pulse-echo ultrasound equipment; a survey of powers pressures and intensities *Brit J Radiol* 58 989–1001
5 FARMERY M J and WHITTINGHAM T A 1978 A portable radiation-force balance for use with diagnostic ultrasound equipment *Ultrasound in Med & Biol* 3 373–379
6 PRESTON R C, BACON D R, LIVETT A J and RAJENDRAN K, 1983 PVDF membrane hydrophone performance properties and their relevance to the measurement of the acoustic output of medical ultrasonic equipment *J Phys E: Sci Instrum* 16 786–796
7 AMERICAN INSTITUTE of ULTRASOUND in MEDICINE/NATIONAL ELECTRICAL MANUFACTURERS ASSOCIATION (AIUM/NEMA), 1983 Safety standard for diagnostic ultrasound equipment, UL 1–1981 *J Ultrasound in Med* 2 (*Suppl*)
8 STARRITT H C and DUCK F A 1986 The dependence of measured beam parameters on power (Proceedings of this Conference: Chapter 8)
9 BACON D R 1984 Finite amplitude distortion of the pulsed fields used in diagnostic ultrasound *Ultrasound in Med & Biol* 10 189–195

CHAPTER 7

Standardisation of Acoustic Output for Diagnostic Ultrasound Equipment—Present and Future

D R Bacon and R C Preston
National Physical Laboratory, Teddington, Middlesex TW11 0LW

7.1 Introduction

The recent concern about the safe use of diagnostic ultrasound imaging in pregnancy[1-3] has led to an increasing awareness of the importance of the standardisation of acoustic output of ultrasound equipment. One of the recommendations of the report by the Royal College of Obstetricians and Gynaecologists (RCOG)[2] notes the lack of beam intensity standards within the United Kingdom, indicates that such a standard should be developed and states that manufacturers should publish intensity values in accordance with it, these values being subject to independent checks. The report recognises that such a standard is a necessary first step if the beam powers used in clinical practice are to be minimised.

This paper discusses the present world position regarding written standards for the specification of ultrasonic output levels, concentrating on the main developments and highlighting the different approaches that are taken to the subject. It is seen that changes have taken place to harmonise the definitions given in the different documents, although there are also suggestions to introduce new and different definitions. The maximum acoustic output levels recommended by the standards are given, and compared with the results of surveys of the measured output levels from equipment. Finally, some of the issues to be resolved in the future are presented along with some conclusions about the present state of knowledge in the subject.

Table 7.1 Published standards.

Organisation	Standard	Date	Origin
AIUM/NEMA	UL1	1981	USA
FDA	510(k)	1984	USA
JSA	JIS T 1503, 4, 5	1984	Japan
IEC	SC 62D (Secretariat)31	1980	International
IEC	SC 29D (Secretariat)26	1985	International

7.2 Published standards

The main published standards are listed in *table 7.1*. The first document mentioned[4] (which was published in 1981) is perhaps the best known and is the result of collaboration between the American Institute for Ultrasound in

55

Medicine and the National Electrical Manufacturers Association (AIUM/NEMA Standard). It gives definitions of the various acoustic parameters, acoustic labelling requirements, guidelines on measurement procedures and a discussion of the safety of ultrasound.

In the USA, the Food and Drug Administration (FDA) has produced several documents, but the most recent and far-reaching one is the 510(k) 'Guide for Measuring and Reporting Acoustic Output of Diagnostic Ultrasound Medical Devices'[5]. This requires manufacturers of new equipment to be sold in the USA to report certain acoustic output parameters to the FDA. The parameters in question are defined and examples are given showing how they should be calculated but, unlike earlier FDA requirements, reference is now made to the AIUM/NEMA Standard for the basic measurement methodology. The principle underlying the document is that equipment should be broadly similar in acoustic output to devices that were available before 1976, and the appropriate 'Pre-Enactment Device Intensities' are given as a reference.

The Japanese Standards Association (JSA) has published several draft standards[6] covering different types of equipment, including a recent draft standard for Electronic Linear Scanning Equipment. Although the main emphasis of these documents is on equipment performance, there are sections covering the measurement of power output and the specification of maximum output levels.

At the international level the International Electrotechnical Commission (IEC) is active in the field of ultrasound standardisation, but all of the documents that deal with diagnostic equipment are still in draft form. IEC Standard Publication 601–2[7] currently requires manufacturers to provide details of certain acoustic output parameters to purchasers for each type of diagnostic equipment sold. A second document[8], provides definitions of a wide range of acoustic parameters, along with the appropriate measurement procedures. This will be a reference for future documents that will define acoustic labelling requirements and, possibly, maximum output levels.

Table 7.2   Status of the standards.

AIUM/NEMA	—Voluntary, to encourage publishing of results.
FDA	—Compulsory, information not published.
JSA	—Draft, mandatory.
IEC	—Draft, would be mandatory in all relevant countries.

One important difference between the different standards is their status, and this information is presented in *table 7.2*. There are currently no standards that compel manufacturers to declare acoustic output levels for diagnostic ultrasound equipment. The Japanese standard JIS T 1504[6] requires the total power output for B-scanning equipment to be stated and there are similar requirements in the corresponding document for linear-array equipment, but these documents are still only in draft form. Nevertheless, information is being made available on the output levels from currently available equipment, either as a result of the voluntary AIUM/NEMA Standard[4] (and the AIUM commendation scheme), or as a result of independent measurements[9], or in a non-specific form as a result of information supplied to the FDA[10].

7.3 Differences between standards

Apart from their status, the most important differences between the standards are their general methods of approach, in terms of the measuring devices that are specified and the types of parameter that are defined. The measuring devices that are commonly specified are hydrophones (to measure the spatial and temporal characteristics of fields) and radiation pressure balances (to measure total power). If hydrophones are used, then the measured parameters can be defined in terms of intensity (which is assumed to be proportional to the square of the acoustic pressure) or acoustic pressure. The IEC standards prefer the latter approach, because acoustic pressure is the field parameter that is actually measured by a hydrophone, whereas the other standards specify intensity parameters. The Japanese standards specify intensity in terms of total power divided by the radiating area of the transducer, whereas the American Standards are written in terms of hydrophone and total power measurements.

Since the Japanese standards are radically different in approach from the three other documents dealing with diagnostic equipment, they will not be discussed further in this section. Setting aside the methods of approach, there were until recently two main differences in the definitions of acoustic parameters. The standards defined the pulse duration and the beam area in different ways, and this gave rise to differences in the definitions for the spatial-average and pulse-average parameters. Now however, the 510(k) document, which has recently been introduced by the FDA, and the most recent revision of the IEC standard[8] are in agreement with the definitions of the AIUM/NEMA Standard. Although there is currently a general consensus about the definitions of acoustic parameters, there have recently been suggestions that the temporal-peak intensity should be defined in a different way[11]. The suggestions are based on the fact that it is often difficult to measure the true peak intensity and the opinion that it would be easier to measure the intensity averaged over the largest half-cycle of the acoustic pulse. If such a change were to be proposed, it would probably be difficult to achieve international consensus for the required revisions to the standards.

Table 7.3 Acoustic output parameters to be reported. The symbol X denotes that the parameter should be reported; (X) indicates that the parameter need not be reported for certain types of transducer.

	SPTP Intensity	SPTA Intensity	SPPA Intensity	SATA Intensity	Total Power
AIUM/NEMA		X	X	X	X
FDA	X	X	X	(X)	
JSA				X	
Suggested	X (p_+, p_-)	X			

7.4 Reporting of acoustic parameters

Although many field parameters have been defined, only relatively few have been selected by the standards for reporting or acoustic output labelling requirements. These parameters are indicated in *table 7.3*, where the following four intensity parameters are included: spatial-peak temporal-peak (SPTP) intensity, spatial-peak temporal-average (SPTA) intensity, spatial-peak pulse-average (SPPA)

57

intensity and spatial-average temporal-average (SATA) intensity. In general, these parameters are defined in the focal region of the radiating transducer, but some standards define the spatial average intensity in terms of acoustic power divided by transducer area, as discussed above. A minimum set of acoustic parameters has been suggested at the National Physical Laboratory as indicated in the bottom row of the table. It is suggested that the SPTP parameter should be defined in terms of the peak-positive and peak-negative acoustic pressures (p_+ and p_- respectively). These parameters are thought to be important because the negative pressure may be relevant to the possible occurrence of cavitation damage whereas the positive pressure usually has the greatest magnitude. The SPTA intensity is included because it is relevant to possible thermal effects.

Table 7.4 Acoustic output levels mentioned in the standards.

	SPTP Intensity (W cm^{-2})	SPTA Intensity (mW cm^{-2})	SPPA Intensity (W cm^{-2})	SATA (power/area) (mW cm^{-2})
AIUM/NEMA		100		
FDA (general)	1700	170	240	20
(highest)	1700	920	240	380
JSA				10
IEC	?	?	?	?

Table 7.5 Acoustic output levels from diagnostic equipment[9, 12]. The asterisks denote values that exceed the appropriate levels given in *table 7.4*.

	SPTP Intensity (W cm^{-2})	SPTA Intensity (mW cm^{-2})	SPPA Intensity (W cm^{-2})
Static pulse-echo scanners[9]	280–2800*	19–180*	36–1100*
Automatic sector scanners[9]	300–3700*	24–680*	33–320*
Linear arrays[9]	0.7–1000	0.07–2.5	0.4–130
Continuous-wave doppler[12]		20–800*	

Specific maximum levels for certain parameters are mentioned in the standards and these are presented in *table 7.4*. The FDA specify different acoustic levels for devices with different applications, so the levels for general scanning equipment are given separately from the highest level given for any equipment type. The IEC has not yet specified any acoustic output levels, but a new working group is now being set up to study this possibility (SC 29D, WG11).

For comparison purposes, *table 7.5* gives the results of a recent survey of output levels from diagnostic equipment[9], where the asterisks denote a value that exceeds the maximum level given in at least one of the standards. None of the data for linear-array scanners exceeds any of the specified maximum levels, whereas the data for the other types of equipment exceed these levels for each of the parameters measured. It should be noted here that the data for continuous-wave doppler devices were obtained from a different source (*reference 12*: p 65). These observations support the view that only a few parameters are necessary to characterise equipment, since the maximum output parameters for each type of equipment either all exceed the specified levels or are all less than these levels.

7.5 Conclusion

Three conclusions can be drawn from this paper, namely that there is now an international consensus about the definition of the important acoustic field parameters for the characterisation of diagnostic ultrasound equipment, that some equipment currently available exceeds the maximum output levels that have been specified, and that only a few parameters may serve to characterise equipment.

Two issues have still to be decided at the IEC level, and are therefore of interest to member nations such as the United Kingdom. These are the possible definition of acoustic labelling requirements and the specifications of maximum acoustic output levels.

References

1   US DEPARTMENT OF HEALTH AND HUMAN SERVICES, NATIONAL INSTITUTES OF HEALTH 1984 *Diagnostic Ultrasound Imaging in Pregnancy.* NIH Publication No 84–667 (US Government Printing Office, Washington, DC 20402)
2   ROYAL COLLEGE OF OBSTETRICIANS AND GYNAECOLOGISTS 1984 *Report of the RCOG working party on routine ultrasound examination in pregnancy* (Royal College of Obstetricians and Gynaecologists, 27 Sussex Place, Regents Park, London NW1 4RG)
3   JAPANESE SOCIETY OF ULTRASONICS IN MEDICINE 1984 On the views on safety of diagnostic ultrasound *Ultrasound in Med & Biol* **10** 556–571
4   AIUM/NEMA 1981 *Safety standard for diagnostic ultrasound equipment* Publication UL 1–1981, (National Electrical Manufacturers Association, 2101 L Street NW, Washington DC 20037, USA)
5   US FOOD AND DRUG ADMINISTRATION 1984 *Guide for measuring and reporting acoustic output of diagnostic ultrasound medical devices* (Draft) Document 510(k) (Center for Devices and Radiological Health, HFZ–132, Rockville MD 20857, USA)
6   JAPANESE STANDARDS ASSOCIATION 1984 *Japanese Industrial Standards JIS T 1503, JIS T 1504 and JIS T 1505* (Japanese Standards Association, 1–24 Akasaka 4-chome, Minato-ku, Tokyo 107)
7   INTERNATIONAL ELECTROTECHNICAL COMMISSION 1980 *Ultrasonic medical diagnostic equipment, part 2. Particular requirements for safety* IEC Standard 601–2–IEC/SC 62D (Secretariat)
8   INTERNATIONAL ELECTROTECHNICAL COMMISSION 1985 *Measurement and characterisation of ultrasonic fields using hydrophones in the frequency range 0.5 MHz to 15 MHz* IEC/SC 29D (Secretariat)26
9   DUCK F A, STARRITT H C, AINDOW J D, PERKINS M A and HAWKINS A J 1985 The output of pulse-echo ultrasound equipment; a survey of powers, pressures and intensities *Brit J Radiol* **58** 989–1001
10 STEWART H F 1983 Output levels from commercial diagnostic ultrasound equipment *J Ultrasound in Med* **2** (10) 39
11 NATIONAL COUNCIL ON RADIATION PROTECTION AND MEASUREMENTS 1983 *Biological effects of ultrasound: mechanisms and clinical implications* NCRP Report No 74 (NCRP, Bethesda, MD 20814, USA)
12 WORLD HEALTH ORGANISATION 1982 *Environmental Health Criteria 22, Ultrasound* (WHO, Geneva)

CHAPTER 8

The Dependence of Measured Beam Parameters on Power

H C Starritt and F A Duck
Medical Physics Department, Royal United Hospital, Bath BA1 3NG

8.1 Introduction

The correct measurement of several standard parameters used to characterise focused beams from diagnostic ultrasonic equipment depends upon the ability to accurately locate the position of the focus. This paper discusses the problems of attempting to locate the focal zone of a focused transducer using only a membrane hydrophone.

The first problem is the definition of focal length which may be surprisingly complex. The AIUM/NEMA standard[1] defines FOCAL LENGTH as the distance along the beam axis of a focusing transducer assembly to the focal surface. The FOCAL SURFACE is defined as the surface which contains the smallest of all beam cross-sectional areas and the BEAM CROSS-SECTIONAL AREA is defined as the area on the surface of a plane, perpendicular to the beam axis, consisting of all points where the pulse intensity integral is greater than 25 per cent of the maximum pulse intensity integral in that plane.

So, at the focus the beam cross-sectional area is a minimum but in order to measure that area correctly it is necessary to calculate the pulse intensity integral for all points on a surface perpendicular to the transducer.

8.2 Pulse intensity integral

If a waveform is continuous and sinusoidal the time averaged intensity, I, can be calculated from the value of peak pressure, $\hat{p}$, using the expression

$$I = \frac{\hat{p}^2}{2\rho c}$$

However for pulses, this formula cannot be applied and it is usual to calculate a pulse-average intensity from the pulse intensity integral.
The pulse intensity integral is defined as:

$$\frac{1}{\rho c} \int_0^t p^2 dt$$

and the pulse average intensity is obtained by dividing this by the pulse length. We have used the AIUM definition of pulse length which is $1.25 \times$ the time between 10 per cent and 90 per cent on the intensity integral curve. One problem with the practical application of this definition is that the pulse length measured is critically dependent on the location of the thresholds in relation to the shape of the pulse intensity integral curve.

The use of pulse intensity integral as the parameter defining the location of the focus initially appears clumsy and inconvenient and it may seem that the peak pressure detected by a hydrophone could be used more simply to locate the focus of a beam. We have investigated the consequences of doing so and deducing standard beam parameters from measurements made, not at the true focus of a beam, but at the position of maximum pressure.

8.3   Experimental measurements

In the experiments described here a 3.5 MHz transducer (KB–Aerotech QSB 35DM) and a Fisher Diasonograph 4200 static B scanner were used. The transducer was 13 mm in diameter and had a stated focal zone of 4 to 10 cm. The variable transmit attenuation control on the Diasonograph allowed the pressure at

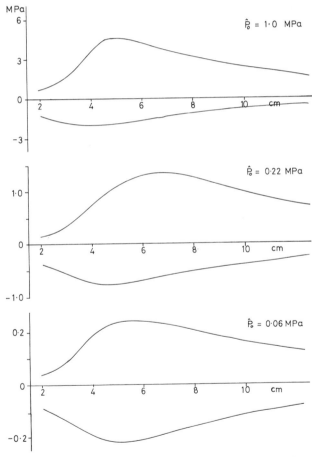

Figure 8.1   Longitudinal plot of peak axial pressure against distance from a focused transducer for three input pressures, $\hat{p}_o$
f = 3.5 MHz d = 13 mm

the transducer to be varied over a wide range and this pressure (measured by positioning a hydrophone immediately adjacent to the transducer) could be varied from approximately 1.0 MPa to 0.02 MPa. The effects described have also been observed with two different transducers viz, a 2.25 MHz, 19 mm diameter, 9 cm focus and a 5 MHz, 13 mm diameter, 5–12 cm focus.

The measurements were made in distilled water using a 9 μm coplanar hydrophone coupled to a Tektronix 465 oscilloscope with the bandwidth limited to 20 MHz. This hydrophone was cross-calibrated against a 2 × 25 μm bilaminar hydrophone having an NPL calibration. This was done by accurately positioning both hydrophones in turn in the beam and recording the peak pressures measured over a range of output powers. It was noted to be essential when making measurements with the coplanar screened hydrophone that the hydrophone is immersed to a constant depth in the water since any drop in the water level below the top of the membrane produces an increase in the observed voltage.

For each of the three transducers longitudinal plots of maximum positive and maximum negative pressure, on the beam axis, over a range of 2–13 cm from the transducer were made. The pressure was measured at 2 mm steps for nine different values of input pressure.

Figure 8.1 shows three such longitudinal plots at input pressures of 1.0, 0.2 and 0.06 MPa. The position of the peak positive pressure can be seen to vary with power. For this particular combination of transducer and driver the peak positive pressure is located closer to the transducer at maximum and minimum powers than at intermediate powers. The shift in location is less marked for the negative pressure peaks where there is a steady move towards the transducer as the power increases.

For each of the nine input pressures a 'zone of maximum pressure' was defined as the region in which the pressure was within 0.5 dB of the maximum pressure and the location of this region, in terms of distance from the transducer, was recorded from the longitudinal plots.

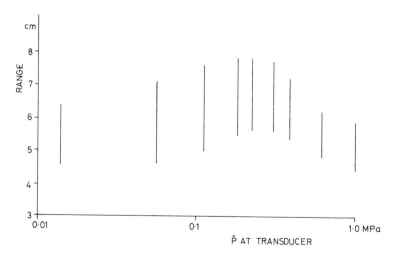

Figure 8.2 Location of zone of maximum positive pressure against input pressure, $\hat{p}_0$
Transducer as *figure 8.1*

Figure 8.2 combines the results of the nine individual plots. The horizontal axis represents the input pressure and the vertical axis is distance from the transducer. The length of the lines represents the extent of the maximum pressure zones as described above and their position represents the relative locations with reference to the transducer. Again the high and low power pressure maxima occur closer to the transducer than for intermediate powers.

Figure 8.3 is a similar plot showing the locations of the peak negative pressure zones. As shown before there is a steady shift towards the transducer as the power increases. The effect is less marked than in the case of positive pressure but nevertheless a shift in location of the peak occurred.

The shift in the location of peak pressure is thought to occur as a result of a combination of finite amplitude effects and diffraction effects in focused fields. At low power finite amplitude effects are unimportant, but as the power increases the wave begins to crest-up progressively through and beyond the focus, so that the pressure peak occurs beyond the low amplitude focus. At very high power levels cresting occurs earlier, before the true focus, but acoustic saturation effects come into play so that the pressure peak is located closer to the transducer.

The difference in the location of the positive and negative peaks at any one output power can be explained by considering the changes in pulse shape which occur during propagation. The photographs in *figure 8.4* were taken at 1 cm intervals along the beam axis. We can see that as the pulse propagates it becomes increasingly asymmetric, with the positive pressure peak becoming much greater in magnitude than the negative pressure peak. A series of photographs such as these was made for each of three output powers and were digitised by hand using a Commodore PET and a digitising pad in order to calculate the pulse intensity integral and the pulse length for each pulse.

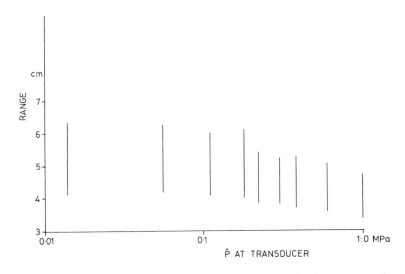

Figure 8.3   Location of zone of maximum negative pressure against input pressure, $\hat{p}_0$
Transducer as *figure 8.1*

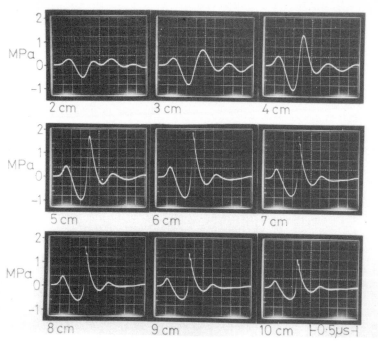

Figure 8.4 Variation in pulse shape with propagation distance from the transducer
$\dot{P}_0 = 300$ kPa
Transducer as *figure 8.1*

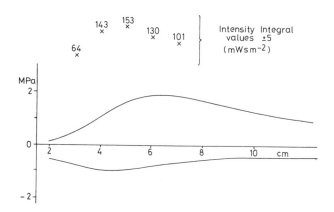

Figure 8.5 Comparison of the location of maximum pulse intensity integral and maximum peak pressure at constant input pressure.

Figure 8.5 shows five values of pulse intensity integral superimposed on a longitudinal plot of axial pressure for one input pressure. It can be seen that the pulse intensity integral peaks at a different range from the transducer than does the positive pressure (the negative pressure peak is closer). This comparison was carried out at three input pressures—0.6, 0.3 and 0.06 MPa and in each case the pulse measured at 5 cm resulted in the maximum value of pulse intensity integral whilst the location of the peak pressure measurement varied. At the minimum power the peak pressure measurement also occurred at about 5 cm. These results indicate that the location of the pulse intensity integral is less dependent on input power than is the location of peak pressure.

Pressure profiles were measured at 0.5 cm intervals along the beam axis for four different input powers with input pressures varying from 0.6–0.06 MPa. The −6 dB beam diameter at each location was measured. *Figure 8.6* shows plots of the variation in beam diameters with range. The positive pressure beam diameters are represented by solid lines and the negative pressure beam diameters by broken lines. In each case the minimum beam diameter occurs at approximately 5 cm from the transducer. Plotted on these graphs also are the location of the peak positive pressure zones and peak negative pressure zones, varying with power, as previously described. From these plots it is very clear that measuring the beam

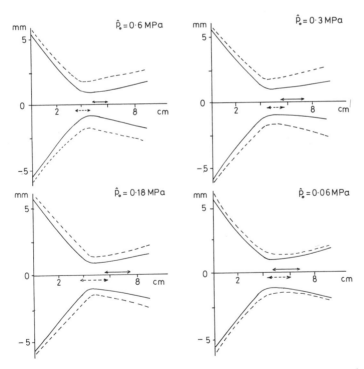

Figure 8.6   Location of minimum beam diameters and maximum pressure zones for input pressures in the range 0.06–0.6 MPa. (Solid lines represent positive pressure measurements, broken lines represent negative pressure measurements).

diameter at the position of peak pressure will lead to an over-estimate of the beam cross-sectional area for a radially symmetric transducer. The problem is much more complex for an astigmatic focusing system.

8.4 Conclusions

From these measurements and within the limits of the experiments it is concluded that location of maximum pulse intensity integral and minimum beam cross-sectional area are not strongly dependent on input power. On the other hand we have shown conclusively for three separate medical transducers that the location of the peak pressure changes with the input power and cannot therefore be generally used as an indicator of focal location. Measurements made with a hydrophone at this location will underestimate spatial peak, temporal average and pulse average intensities and gain, and will overestimate beam cross-sectional area. Furthermore, the location of spatial peak temporal peak intensity (calculated from $\hat{p}^2/\rho c$) does not coincide with the location of spatial peak pulse average intensity or spatial peak temporal average intensity (both calculated from the pulse intensity integral).

Whilst it is possible to locate the focal zone by peak pressure measurements when the output power is low, many clinical pulse-echo systems operate only in the 'shifted' region[2]. It will be important therefore to develop measurement systems which give pulse intensity integral and intensity directly, if accurate dosimetry is to be carried out.

References

1 AMERICAN INSTITUTE OF ULTRASOUND IN MEDICINE/NATIONAL ELECTRICAL MANUFACTURERS ASSOCIATION (AIUM/NEMA), 1983 Safety standard for diagnostic ultrasound equipment, UL 1–1981 *J Ultrasound in Med 2* (Suppl)
2 DUCK F A, STARRITT H C, AINDOW J D, PERKINS M A and HAWKINS A J 1985 The output of pulse-echo ultrasound equipment; a survey of powers, pressures and intensities *Brit J Radiol* **58** 989–1001

CHAPTER 9

Practical Beamshapes as Visualised by the Newcastle Beam Plotting System

T A Whittingham and T J Roberts
*Regional Medical Physics Department, Newcastle General Hospital,
Newcastle-upon-Tyne NE4 6BE*

9.1 Introduction

This paper presents examples of the spatial pressure distributions (beamplots) in the axial and transverse planes of some ultrasonic transducers and comments on their principal features. The field structure revealed by these plots assists in the understanding and teaching of the underlying diffraction theory. They also provide useful quantitative information about the lateral resolving capability and safety-related intensity and pressure characteristics of medical imaging equipment. Attention is drawn to the inappropriate use of the terms near-field and far-field when describing focused beams.

9.2 Brief system description

The beam plots presented here were produced by an automated beam plotting system designed and built within the Department[1]. A full account of the system will be published shortly, but essentially it consists of a tank of water in which a piezoelectric hydrophone is driven in any required vertical or horizontal plane under the control of an Apple II microcomputer. The transducer under examination is coupled to the water tank by a thin plastic membrane in a side wall. The measured pressure distribution in the selected plane is presented as either a colour or grey scale real-time display. It is also stored for further processing or reference on the Apple's floppy magnetic disc. Measurement of either continuous wave pressure amplitude or peak pulse pressure amplitude is possible. Substitution of a reflective target allows pulse-echo sensitivity plots to be made as a means of assessing the effective beam shape resulting from signal processing in reception. Measurement of a particular beam from a free running real-time probe may be made by strobing a receiver gate once per real-time frame. A typical plot consisting of a matrix of 100 by 100 sample points takes approximately 5 minutes to complete.

Although the system is capable of measuring absolute pressures using a calibrated hydrophone, the grey scales marked on the plots shown here are on a relative scale of 0 to 255. The points at which the pressure reaches the plot maximum of 255 are indicated by black dots within the surrounding peak white. Each grey level, with the exception of the lowest level, represents a range of 6 dB.

9.3 Comparison of cw and peak-detected plots

Figure 9.1 shows the pressure distribution in an axial plane for an 18 mm diameter transducer with a nominal frequency of 2.25 MHz and a nominal focal length of

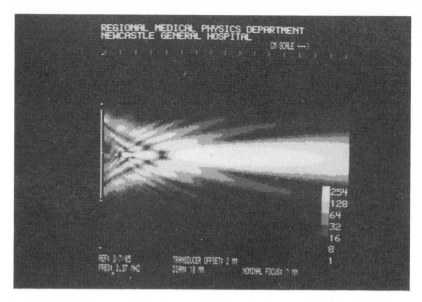

Figure 9.1a Continuous wave (cw) longitudinal beam plot of an 18 mm diameter, 2.37 MHz transducer having a geometric focal length of 115 mm.

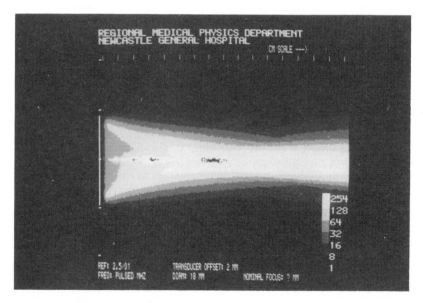

Figure 9.1b Peak-detected beam plot of the same transducer as in *figure 9.1a* operated in a shock-excited pulsed mode.

115 mm. *Figure 9.1a* is for continuous wave (cw) excitation, and *figure 9.1b* is for pulsed excitation with the displayed quantity being the peak amplitude of the full-wave rectified pulse. As expected, the diffraction maxima and minima are more pronounced for the monochromatic case than for the wide bandwidth pulse, but the overall beam shapes, as defined by, say, the 18 dB contour, are fairly similar. The characteristics of focused beams will be discussed in the following section, but for the moment we shall compare the two plots.

The diffraction pattern in the cw case is the result of integration across the full aperture. For the pulsed case the pattern may be considered to be the result of interference between two pulses: a plane pulse wave parallel to the transducer face and extending between the lateral limits of the transducer's geometric shadow, and an edge pulse wave radiating from a line source around the transducer periphery. If we consider a simplification of the transducer as a straight line source within the scan plane, we can consider the cw pattern as the summation of contributions from all points along the line, and the pulsed case as the summation of a direct wave and a point source at each end of the line. An important feature of the edge pulse waves is that they have the same polarity as the direct wave where their initial direction is outside the geometric shadow, but they are inverted where this is inside the geometric shadow.

This simple line source model would predict that axial maxima should occur at similar ranges for both cw and pulsed plots, since for both cases an axial maximum requires that the difference in path length between contributions from the centre and the periphery of the transducer should be an odd number of half wavelengths. The practical beam plots shown here support this prediction. The variation of pressure across the beam is much smoother for the pulsed case, with beam profiles having generally flatter tops. Exceptions to this occur at those ranges which correspond to axial maxima as, for a pulsed beam, these are shaped like very pronounced and narrow fins on an otherwise flat crest. The flat top of the beam may be explained by considering the temporal separation between the three pulses of the line source model. A peak detector output will simply correspond to the largest of the three pulses, since for most positions within the beam there will be no overlap of pulses. The overlap that is necessary for the production of maxima will only occur on or close to the axis, so their lateral extent will be small.

Important considerations for peak-detected plots are whether the rectification is full wave or half wave, whether it acts on an inverted or non-inverted pulse, and the polarity and shape of the acoustic pulse. Thus a particular maximum might be demonstrated with full-wave rectification but would be missing with half-wave rectification having the opposite polarity to the reinforced half cycle. It is also possible for some potential maxima to be lost due to the dominant effect of a large half cycle in a pulse with an irregular or strongly damped shape. Apart from such diffraction effects, non-linear propagation effects cause the amplitude of positive half cycles to exceed those of negative half cycles, with the result that the positions of diffraction maxima and minima would depend on the polarity of the detection system (see Starritt and Duck, Chapter 8).

9.4 Focused beams

Inspection of *figure 9.1a* shows that a focused beam consists of three distinguishable regions:

(a)   A focal zone, where the lateral width of the beam is a minimum and the axial amplitude is a maximum. A transverse beam profile within the region has the same $J_1(x)/x$ function that is characteristic of the far-field of an unfocused probe. ($J_1(x)$ is Bessel's function of the first kind). In general the amplitude distribution in the focal plane (or at a large range in the far-field of an unfocused probe) is the Fourier Transform of that in the transducer aperture. This relationship, which is characteristic of Fraunhofer diffraction, is a consequence of the linear increase in path length with distance across the transducer. In the reception mode this is equivalent to saying that curvature of the waveform from a point in the focal zone closely matches that of the transducer.

The beam and side-lobe structure in the focal zone will therefore be conical with the same angles as those in the far-field of an unfocused transducer of the same diameter and frequency. The first off-axis nulls predicted by the $J_1(x)/x$ expression may be seen extending for the length of the focal zone. These nulls could be called Fraunhofer nulls. At the range (R) of the geometric focus, this predicts a beamwidth measured between nulls of 1.2 λR/a for a disc transducer, where λ is wavelength and a is the transducer radius. This agrees with the width as measured from *figure 9.1a*.

The point of maximum axial amplitude is seen to be displaced towards the transducer from the geometric focus. This is due to the inverse relationship between the amplitude of a contribution from a point of the transducer and the path length to the field point. At the axial peak the gain in amplitude due to the decrease in range more than compensates for the decrease resulting from the slight differences between the path lengths of contributions from differing points. The same effect is responsible for the existence of an axial peak in amplitude (and a comensurate decrease in beamwidth) at the near-field to far-field transition of an unfocused transducer.

A theoretical analysis predicts that the range (F) of the axial peak is equal to p.R, where R is the geometric focal length and p is a factor that depends on the strength of focusing. Defining $D = a^2/\lambda$ as the length of the near-field of the equivalent unfocused transducer having the same wavelength (λ) and radius (a), the value of p decreases approximately linearly from 0.99 to 0.60 as R/D increases from 0.1 to 1.0. For the case shown in *figure 9.1a*, where R/D = 0.88 (p = 0.64), this theory predicts an axial peak at 74 mm, agreeing with the observed position on the beam plot.

(b)   A region between the transducer and the focal zone which exhibits diffraction maxima and minima. This is contained approximately within the geometric shadow of the transducer, taking the form of a cone with the transducer aperture as its base and the geometric focus as its apex. This zone is analogous to the near-field of an unfocused transducer, since the conditions for maxima and minima depend on path differences in precisely the same way as for an unfocused transducer. In fact, amplitude variations within this zone may be predicted from those within the near-field of an unfocused transducer of the same frequency and diameter by a transformation in which coordinates perpendicular and parallel to the axis of the unfocused transducer are replaced by a bearing and a range parameter centred on the geometric focus[3].

(c)   A region beyond the focal zone where further diffraction effects may occur. In the weakly focused example of *figure 9.1a* the only clear evidence of this is the termination of the first off-axis nulls near the right edge of the beamplot. *Figure 9.2* shows the beam from a much more strongly focused transducer (R/D = 0.056) and here two further axial maxima may be seen beyond the focal zone. This region is also approximately contained within the cone of the geometric

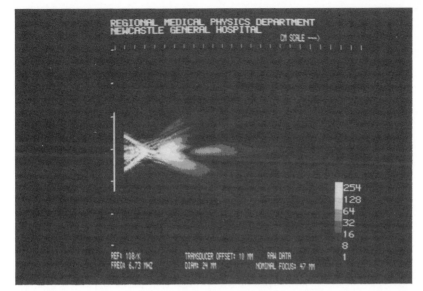

Figure 9.2 Continuous wave longitudinal beam plot of a strongly focused transducer: diameter 24 mm; frequency 6.73 MHz; nominal geometric focal length 37 mm.

shadow lying beyond the geometric focus. The diffraction effects in this region may also be obtained by a transformation of the diffraction pattern of the near-field of the equivalent unfocused transducer.

The regions proximal and distal to the focal zone are caused by the same diffraction effects that produce the near-field of an unfocused transducer. In a reception mode these can be summarised by saying that the wavefront curvature is significantly different to that of a simple bowl transducer having its centre of curvature at the geometric focus.

Clearly, as there are three regions in a focused beam, the notion of a near-field and a far-field is inappropriate. It is therefore proposed that the terms near-field and far-field be restricted to unfocused beams and that other names be used for the three regions of a focused beam. Possible names for the three zones described above might be those proposed previously[3], being respectively:

(a)   near Fresnel zone
(b)   focal zone (or Fraunhofer zone)
(c)   far Fresnel zone

9.5   Multi-element transducer arrays

A linear array of narrow rectangular elements, each element approximating to a line source, may be used to step a beam sideways to give a linear scan, or to steer a beam about a central element to give a sector scan. Commercial real-time scanners employing these techniques are popularly known as 'linear array' and 'phased array' systems respectively, although stepped array and steered array would be more descriptive names. In a typical stepped array a group of, say 10 adjacent

71

elements, forms the active transducer area, with an element width of say 3 wavelengths. The scan is made by advancing this group along an array of say 64 elements. In a typical steered array of say 64 elements, the element spacing will be approximately 0.5 wavelengths and all the elements will contribute to each beam.

In the following discussion the convention will be followed that describes distances or dimensions within the scan plane, but perpendicular to the beam axis, as azimuthal and those perpendicular to the scan plane as elevational.

The beams from rectangular arrays differ from those of the simple disc transducers used in A-mode, M-mode or mechanically scanned real-time scanners in three ways, as demonstrated in *figure 9.3* which shows beam cross-sections at various ranges for a commercial stepped array:

(a)   The shape of the beam cross-section varies with range, from rectangular close to the transducer (*figure 9.3a*), through a cross shape in the focal region (*figures 9.3b to 9.3c*), to a generally elliptical shape beyond the focal region (*figure 9.3d*). In the example of *figure 9.3a*, where a short transmission focal length has been selected, the active transducer area is narrower in azimuth than in elevation; for longer transmission focal lengths more elements would be used, giving a more square aperture. Slight variations in output between the individual elements are also apparent, but no evidence of deliberate apodization (amplitude shading) is apparent.

The cross shape in the focal zone is a consequence of the previously mentioned Fourier Transform relationship that exists between the amplitude distribution in the plane of the transducer aperture and that in the focal plane.

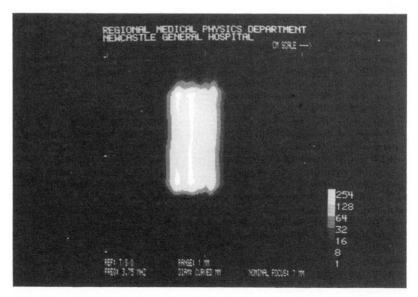

Figure 9.3a   Transverse section of a peak-detected beam plot at a range of 1 mm from a commercial linear array probe: frequency 3.75 MHz; focal length in plane of azimuth 28 mm; focal length in plane of elevation 50 mm.

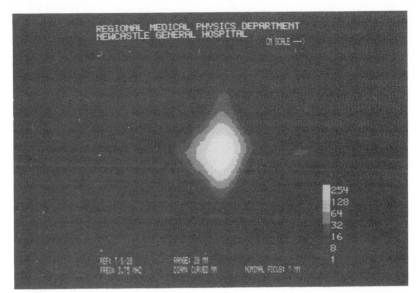

Figure 9.3b Transverse section of the same beam at the range of the azimuthal focus (28 mm range).

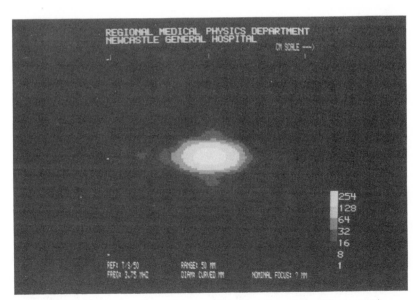

Figure 9.3c Transverse section at the range of the elevational focus (50 mm range).

73

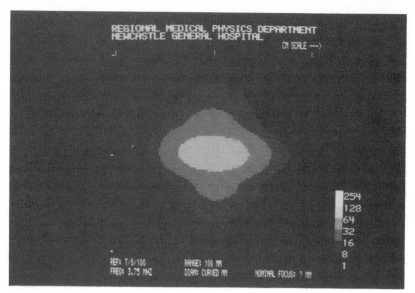

Figure 9.3d Transverse section at a range of 100 mm.

(b)   The variation of beamwidth with range, and the range of minimum beamwidth are likely to be different in azimuth and elevation since beamwidth characteristics in elevation are determined by a fixed lens, whilst those in the scan plane may be varied electronically either by the operator or dynamically according to pre-programmed sequences (so-called dynamic aperture and dynamic-focus techniques). In the example shown in *figure 9.3*, a short azimuthal focal length (28 mm) has been selected, whereas the fixed elevational focal length is 50 mm. As a consequence of these different focal lengths this beam has no single focal plane where the amplitude is the 2D Fourier Transform of the transducer aperture. Instead there is a 1D Fourier Transform relationship between the aperture function in azimuth and the beam profile in azimuth at the azimuthal focal range, and a 1D Fourier Transform relationship between the aperture function in elevation and the beam profile in elevation at the elevational focal range. The main lobe of this beam is therefore narrower in azimuth than in elevation at the azimuthal focus (*figure 9.3b*) but is wider in azimuth than in elevation at the elevational focus (*figure 9.3c*).

(c)   There may be grating lobes in the scan plane caused by constructive interference between adjacent elements of the array. They will be almost eliminated if the centre-to-centre element spacing is less than half a wavelength. This condition is satisfied in some recent steered arrays, but it is unlikely to be satisfied in stepped arrays. The latter are therefore subject to significant acoustic noise owing to spurious off-axis echoes from the grating lobes. These lobes are clearly visible in *figure 9.4* which shows a peak-detected plot of a 'linear array' probe, obtained by stroboscopically sampling the output from the hydrophone after the same transmission in each frame. Their amplitude relative to the main lobe is determined by the directivity of a single element, being, in theory, zero for

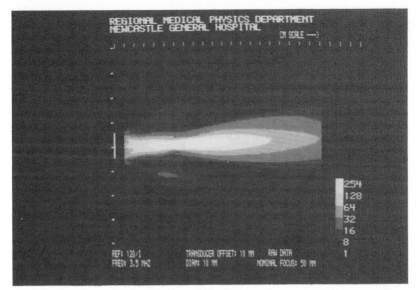

Figure 9.4 Longitudinal section of a peak detected beam plot of a 3.5 MHz commercial linear array probe, demonstrating grating lobes.

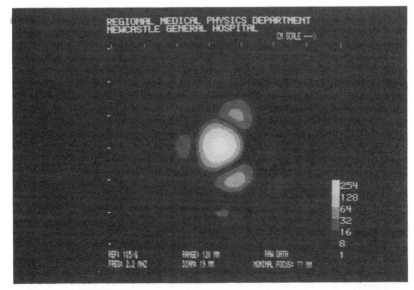

Figure 9.5 Transverse section at a range of 120 mm through the cw beam plot from a suspect 2.2 MHz, 19 mm diameter unfocused transducer, demonstrating asymmetrical side-lobe structure.

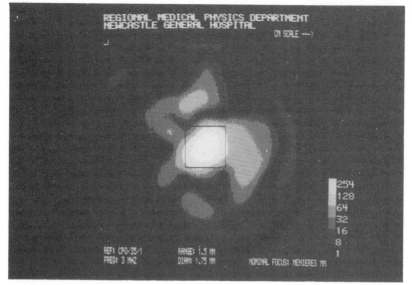

Figure 9.6   Transverse section at a range of 1.5 mm through the cw beamplot of a surgical probe: transmitting aperture 3.0 mm; frequency 3 MHz.

an array having an inter-element gap of zero width, to –20 dB for a gap of ten per cent of the element width. Electronic deflection of the beam will increase their amplitude dramatically, as demonstrated by the poor performance of early steered arrays in which the half-wavelength spacing criterion was not satisfied[2].

9.6   Examples of applications in quality assurance and dosimetry

Figure 9.5 shows a transverse section through the beam of an unfocused M-mode transducer near the end of the near-field. This probe had been giving poorer lateral resolution than when new. Although there were no external signs of damage, the unsymmetrical side-lobe pattern indicates a non-uniform sensitivity across the transducer, possibly caused by localised detachment of the backing layer.

Figure 9.6 shows a transverse section through the beam from a 3 MHz probe designed for the surgical treatment of Ménières disease, measured 1.5 mm from the 3 mm diameter radiating aperture. This aperture was slightly irregular, being at the end of the double-walled stainless steel tube which acted as an acoustic waveguide, so it is not surprising to find an asymmetric side-lobe structure. A 1 mm square has been superimposed by the computer. Summation of the squares of the amplitudes in each pixel by the computer shows that 73 per cent of the total power of the beam at this range lies within this square.

9.7   Conclusion

Longitudinal and transverse beam plots have a useful role in quality assurance and dosimetry. They also provide a useful experimental basis for a discussion of the theory of beam shapes. Those presented here have illustrated the similarities and differences between continuous wave and peak-detected plots, illustrated the characteristics of beams from array transducers, and have served to demonstrate the desirability of adopting alternatives to the terms near-field and far-field when discussing focused beams. The terms *near-Fresnel zone, focal zone* (or *Fraunhofer zone*), and *far-Fresnel zone* have been proposed.

Acknowledgement

We would like to thank Professor K Boddy for his support of this work, and to gratefully acknowledge the contributions made by Mr I Palmer and Dr K Martin and Mr M Feeney to the design and construction of the beam plotting system. We would like to thank Mr C P Oates for providing the beam plot of *figure 9.6.*

References

1   ROBERTS T J, WHITTINGHAM T A and FEENEY M 1982 A microcomputer controlled beam plotting system *HPA Workshop on Medical Ultrasonic Transducers*, London, 8th October, 1982
2   WHITTINGHAM T A 1981 Real-time ultrasonic scanning *Physical Aspects of Medical Imaging*, Editors Moores B M, Parker R P and Pullan B R, (John Wiley and Sons)
3   WHITTINGHAM T A 1983 Beam shapes from focussed transducers—a conceptual discussion *HPA Conference 'Physics in Medical Ultrasound'*, Hatfield College, Durham, 7–8th July 1983

CHAPTER 10

A Versatile Schlieren System for Beam and Wavefront Visualisation with Quantitative Real-Time Profiling Capability

D H Follett
Medical Physics Department, Bristol General Hospital, Bristol BS1 6SP

10.1 Introduction

The schlieren technique has a long history and at Bristol has been in use for about 25 years [1]. Indeed, some of the original components are used in the present system. It does not, however, seem to have been popular with medical physicists, being largely confined to acoustic research laboratories and educational establishments. In the past this has perhaps been due to supposed practical difficulties or because the method has been considered non-quantitative.

With modern light sources most of the problems are overcome. For a basic system to visualise continuous wave beam shapes a small quartz-iodine lamp provides plenty of light for projection onto a small screen at life-size. A recent development using cheap light-emitting diodes [2] has revolutionised the stroboscopic visualisation of wavefronts from pulsed transducers, although insufficient light is available for projection in our application. The addition of a high sensitivity television camera overcomes this difficulty and makes for a versatile system since the same LED can be used for both pulse and CW applications and the TV provides flexibility in the choice of recording medium.

However, the use of a TV camera has a much more far reaching outcome. By displaying one or more lines of the video signal on an oscilloscope, single or multiple beam profiles can be obtained, virtually in real-time. Moreover, within limits there is good agreement with profiles obtained using a PVDF hydrophone, although no absolute pressure calibration is possible at present. In the development of transducers for special purposes, such as blood flow measurement, the interactive situation made possible because of the unique real-time capability of schlieren visualisation is greatly enhanced by the addition of quantitative information.

10.2 The optical system

This comprises the classic zig-zag layout as shown schematically in plan view in *figure 10.1*. Light from the LED via condensers C and pin hole P is collimated by concave mirror M_2, and after passing through the test tank is focused onto a stop at S and thus mostly prevented from reaching the viewing system. In *figure 10.1*, a transducer T is shown pointing vertically down. Pressure variations in the beam cause density and refractive index gradients in the water so that the beam acts as a phase contrast diffraction grating and for horizontal wavefronts a vertical diffraction pattern appears on a screen placed at S. The spacing of maxima in the pattern agrees with standard grating theory, but the number of orders visible varies with sound intensity. Thus with continuous waves or long pulses there is a threshold intensity required to refract light into the first order maxima before an

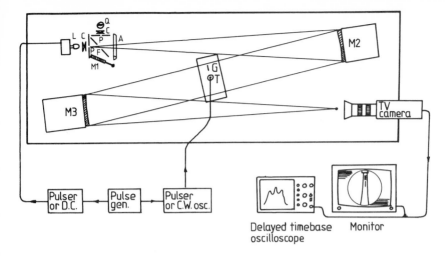

Figure 10.1 Schematic plan of system:

L   Light-emitting diode Stanley H500
C   Condensers, two each 2 cm focal length
P   0.7 mm approx diameter pin hole
F   Beam limit aperture
A   Cylindrical lens 3 dioptres plano-convex
M_1 Front surface plane mirror
Q   50 W quartz iodine lamp
M_2 M_3 150 mm diameter 1220 mm focal length concave telescope mirrors
T   Transducer under test and water tank
G   Graticule
S   Beam stop approx 1.0 mm diameter

image is observable. There is little point making the pinhole image at S much smaller than the spacing of the maxima.

Light from a given point in the ultrasound field is refracted into the diffraction pattern and is then brought to a focus at the imaging plane, mirror M_3 being part of the imaging optics.

A practical problem is that using the mirrors off-axis causes severe astigmatism in the pin hole image at S with about 2 cm separation of vertical (sagittal) and horizontal (tangential) images. In simple systems this is overcome by using, say, the horizontal line image with the stop S being a horizontal line or knife-edge. The result is that vertical wavefronts are not visualised. This means that, for instance, unwanted lateral side lobes from a surgical applicator could be missed which we felt was unacceptable. Accordingly a cylindrical correction lens A is used. There should really be another such lens for M_3 but this would cause severe image distortion requiring further correction. We accept that if the test beam is correctly parallel in the horizontal plane, as in *figure 10.1* then it will not be quite so in the vertical plane. Practically this does not seem to produce any noticeable errors.

When the TV system has been borrowed by colleagues, visualisation of continuous wave beams is still possible using the 50 watt quartz-iodine projector lamp Q housed in a suitable convection chimney to limit stray light. The pivoted

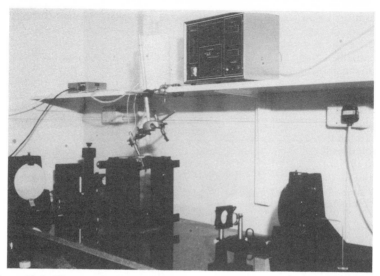

Figure 10.2 Photograph of system. The image projection lens is in position at centre right in place of the TV camera.

plane mirror M_1 is swung over against the aperture F for this purpose. The imaging lens is a simple bi-convex one of about two diopter power, placed close to the stop.

The whole optical system is placed on a 25 mm thick slab of 'bon accord' granite, in turn supported on a rigid steel sub-frame resting on two motor-scooter inner tubes and foam plastic packing. This is not strictly necessary from optical considerations and any flat solid surface would serve; however, it does provide good immunity against changes in weather. The set up is illustrated in *figure 10.2* without the TV system in place, the alternative imaging lens being in position.

10.3 The electronic system

For continuous wave applications, transducers are either excited by their own generators or by an RF oscillator and power amplifier. A calibrated attenuator is also very useful, both for relative calibration purposes and to protect transducers against overload. The LED is supplied with a variable direct current up to about 20 mA. For stroboscopic wavefront visualisation the scheme of *reference 2* is followed, the LED pulser consisting basically of:

(i)   a 74121 TTL Monostable adjustable for 50–250 ns pulse width,
(ii)   a National Semi-conductor DS0026 clock driver operated on 15 V, and
(iii) two IRF 610 MOSFETS (R S Components) with a variable supply about 24–50 V.

The output stage power supply should not be applied suddenly via a switch or the MOSFETS are likely to be destroyed. A supply voltage of 24–30 V is adequate for most uses. The minimum output light pulse width is about 50 ns.

The transducer pulser is similar with a 50–500 ns width adjustment and a single IRF 610 output transistor operating on a fixed 200 V supply. By arranging the transducer pulser for positive edge triggering and the LED pulser for negative edge triggering an ordinary laboratory variable pulse width generator can be used to drive the system, a repetition frequency of about 3000 Hz being suitable. Eventually it is intended to construct a purpose built programmable generator.

On the imaging side the high sensitivity camera feeds a standard 9″ monitor for viewing and recording images onto Polaroid film. A single beam profile at any selected range is displayed on an oscilloscope by connecting the video signal to the Y amplifier. The oscilloscope must have a triggered delayed time base with X magnification capable of locking onto a line sync. pulse. As the time base delay is varied the display then jumps from line to line. In order to determine the range selected various means may be adopted, but the simplest is to recognise the signal from the graticule G (*figure 10.1*). Here again it is intended to build a proper line-counting trigger circuit to give accurate range information and to enable several profiles to be displayed at different ranges simultaneously, thus enabling complete beam characterisation to be obtained in real-time.

10.4 Application, results and discussion

In the stroboscopic mode the usual educational experiments can be made showing generation of plane and edge waves, diffraction, scattering etc. The reversal of phase on reflection at an air-backed membrane may also be nicely illustrated. For

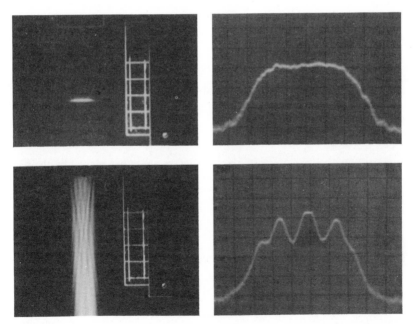

Figure 10.3 Beam profiles under pulse and CW conditions. *Top* Pulse wavefront and profile. Transducer at top. Graticule at left 1 cm squares. At right, horizontal divisions 2.0 mm. *Bottom* CW beam and profile at the same level as the pulse profile.

these visual effects it is usually best to misadjust the stop so that some background illumination is provided, which allows both lighter and darker regions of the wave to show. Better still the stop can be replaced with a corner or a knife edge (if only substantially horizontal wavefronts are to be envisaged), but we do not usually go to this trouble. Beam profiles can be obtained, but it must be remembered that the image represents a narrow slice corresponding with a single TV line and therefore profiles of curved wavefronts occupying more than one TV line are not too meaningful. *Figure 10.3* illustrates profiles and beam visualisation of the same transducer operated under both pulse and continuous wave conditions, and shows how the Fresnel structure present with single frequency CW drive is smoothed out under wider frequency bandwidth pulsed drive.

Quantitative measurements depend on the observation that a graph of peak video output from a profile versus transducer drive voltage is linear over a 20–25 dB range. *Figures 10.4 and 10.5* show comparisons between schlieren profiles and beam plots using a PVDF hydrophone of 1 mm diameter for the same transducer with CW excitations. It is to be expected that the schlieren profile should fall off more rapidly from the peak since refraction of a particular light ray is an integral

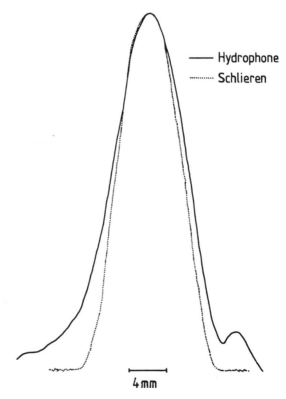

— Hydrophone
········ Schlieren

4 mm

Figure 10.4   Comparison of schlieren and hydrophone beam profiles for a 5 mm diameter PZT unmounted disc, 2.64 MHz and 5 cm range.

effect depending on path length through an ultrasound beam. *Figure 10.4* seems to confirm this for the rather divergent beam whose width at half height is about 8 mm at 5 cm from a transducer only 5 mm diameter. On the other hand, *figure 10.5* shows remarkably good agreement for the much narrower beam resulting from driving the same transducer at its third harmonic. Spatial resolution is basically good, being limited by the TV resolution in our system to about 0.3 mm. The schlieren profiling capability thus appears to be a very useful tool.

There are however a number of limitations to consider. There is no absolute pressure or power calibration although it may be possible to use the spread of the diffraction pattern for this purpose. The system can of course be calibrated for a particular transducer and assumed to be correct for similar ones of the same frequency. The dynamic range of the displays is limited for two reasons. Firstly, there is a threshold of sound intensity as already pointed out which depends on a number of factors such as beam size, shape and frequency. Typically this is around the 10–50 mW cm^{-2} level for continuous waves. It means, for example, that CW Doppler probe beams at 10 MHz can often, but not always, be visualised at normal diagnostic excitation. At high intensities saturation and reverse contrast effects appear, partly due to light being refracted outside the imaging lens, but possibly also due to highly refracted rays interacting with more than one wavefront. The dynamic range between these limits is about 30–35 dB. Secondly, the dynamic range of the TV camera is restricted by noise and saturation to something of the same order, so that the overall linear dynamic range displayed in a profile is not more than 20–25 dB. To some extent this limitation can be circumvented by changing the transducer drive power and using a windowing technique. The TV camera noise is also a problem in itself and makes signal averaging desirable, which so far we have achieved photographically.

Beam alignment in the plane parallel to the light beam is critical for repeatable results, since maximum visualisation occurs when the incident light beam passes parallel to the wavefronts. In connection with this we suspect there are sometimes artefactual beam patterns with highly divergent beams which would not appear on hydrophone plots, but this remains to be confirmed. Certainly anomalous effects might be expected when wavefronts are so curved that a light ray intercepts several in its passage across the sound beam.

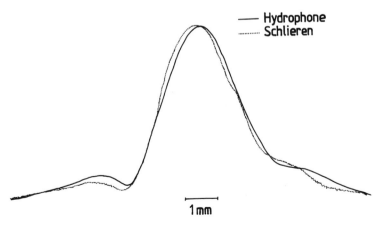

Figure 10.5   As *figure 10.4* but at 8.87 MHz.

83

Finally, there is the lack of portability which is a decided disadvantage for quality control use such as routine checks on physiotherapy transducers. However, for such purposes portability could be achieved by folding the light paths and using only a single concave mirror (or lens). An overall size of about 75 cm by 45 cm by 20 cm is probably a realistic aim for a 15 cm diameter field of view, with the components mounted in a rigid aluminium framework.

References

1   ANGELL JAMES J 1963 New developments in the ultrasonic therapy of Menière's Disease, *Annals of the Royal College of Surgeons* **33** 226–244
2 _ GUNARATHNE G P P and SZILARD J 1983 A new stroboscope for schlieren and photoelectric visualisation of ultrasound, *Ultrasonics* (July) 188–190

Appendix

Components and Suppliers

Main mirrors. Nominal 6.25 inch (158 mm) diameter, 48 inch (1220 mm) focal length $\lambda/8$ low expansion glass telescopic paraboloids available from: David Hinds, 2 Wolsey Road, Hemel Hempstead, Herts HP2 4TU, UK. (Tel 0442–53229). Currently about £100 each, cheaper ones also available.

Glass sides for test tank. At present we use ordinary plate glass which was selected from off-cuts from local glass merchants and cut to size after selection. The glass should be orientated with the striations vertical. Polished plate glass is also available from the above supplier in suitable sizes at about £100 each.

Imaging lens for non-TV applications. Ordinary 35 mm diameter 2D photographic close-up lens.

Condenser lenses about 8 mm diameter, 20 mm focal length. Ex pocket radiation dosimeters.

Astigmation correction lens. Approx 3D (300 mm focal length) Plano-convex 50 mm × 60 mm, Ealing Optics Corp, laboratory quality or similar. Considerable variation in power can be accommodated by position adjustment.

Other optical components, stands etc, Ealing Optics Corp, or similar. The mirror supports are best made in house.

TV Camera. Panasonic WV1850.

Camera Lens. Fujinon TV Zoom Lens C6 × 17.5B (1:1.8/17.5–105). Fuji Photo Optical Co.

LED. Stanley Hi-Super Bright LED type H500, Farnell Electronic components or Lohuis Lamps Ltd. It is advisable to purchase a batch of devices and select those with the most symmetrical beam.

CHAPTER 11

Tissue-Mimicking Materials. A Start Towards their Characterisation

B Zeqiri
National Physical Laboratory, Teddington, Middlesex TW11 0LW

11.1 Introduction

It is generally accepted that the overall performance evaluation of medical ultrasonic equipment would be of clinical benefit. To meet this requirement it has been suggested that materials whose acoustic properties closely resemble those of soft-tissue would be useful to aid the qualitative and quantitative assessment of scanner performance[1]. Consequently, details of the ultrasonic characteristics of suitable materials have been commonplace in the literature[2]. It is also hoped that these materials will have a rôle to play in advanced tissue-characterisation schemes[3]. These aims impose stringent requirements both on material thermal and temporal stability and on available material characterisation techniques. To meet this potential requirement, the NPL has initiated a study into such measurements. Madsen *et al*[4] have suggested that the measurement of ultrasonic attenuation, scatter and velocity as well as medium density provide a suitable set of characterising parameters. One of the aims of this contribution is to invoke participant discussion into what ultrasonic parameters are required to characterise these media, with particular reference to their rôle in providing quality assurance for scanner equipment. For example, at this stage it appears that nonlinear propagation in these media could be important and this needs to be addressed.

As a start to the NPL programme the frequency dependent attenuation coefficient of castor oil has been measured. This has been cited in the literature as a material suitable for the evaluation of experimental technique and procedure[5,6] and for which generally referenced data exists[7].

11.2 Theory

In this study, measurements of the attenuation coefficient of castor oil were made using a through-transmission substitution technique. The experimental arrangement used is depicted schematically in *figure 11.1*. The transmitting transducer is excited by an electrical drive signal at an appropriate frequency, f. Ultrasound propagates through the coupling medium (in this specific case degassed/deionised water) to a receiver located on the acoustic axis of the transducer at a distance z_o from the face of the transducer. The resultant voltage, V_w (f), may be expressed as

$$V_w(f) = R(f) \, U(f) \, \exp(-\alpha_w z_o) \qquad (1)$$

where α_w is the amplitude attenuation coefficient of the carrier medium. The term U(f) relates specifically to the characteristics of the ultrasonic field and it depends on the properties of the particular transmitter and receiver used, as well as on the

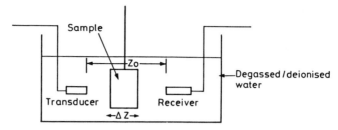

Figure 11.1 Schematic representation of the through-transmission by substitution attenuation coefficient measurement technique.

acoustical parameters of the propagating medium. In contrast, the term $R(f)$ relates to the electrical characteristics of the drive, transduction, detection and amplification circuitry. The parallel-sided sample under investigation is now placed in the path of the ultrasound at a position centred on the acoustic axis with its planar interfaces parallel to the transducer face and the new voltage, $V_s(f)$, recorded. If the sample is of thickness Δz, then

$$V_s(f) = R(f) \exp(-\alpha_w z_0) \exp(-(\alpha_s-\alpha_w)\Delta z) \, t_1 t_2 \, U'(f) \qquad (2)$$

where α_s is the pressure attenuation coefficient of the sample material and t_1 and t_2 represent the amplitude transmission coefficients of the two sample/water interfaces. The displacement, by the sample medium, of an equivalent thickness of water has resulted in a relative attenuation of $\exp(-(\alpha_s-\alpha_w)\Delta z)$. $R(f)$ retains its original meaning, whilst the presence of the sample has now transformed the field dependent term $U(f)$ to $U'(f)$. The amplitude transmission coefficient, $A_s(f)$, may be expressed as

$$A_s(f) = V_s(f)/V_w(f) \qquad (3)$$

which when combined with equations 1 and 2 becomes

$$A_s(f) = \exp(-(\alpha_s-\alpha_w)\Delta z) \, t_1 t_2 \, [U'(f)/U(f)] \qquad (4)$$

By recasting in terms of the intensity and taking logarithms

$$\ln(I_s(f)) = -(\alpha_s^I - \alpha_w^I)\Delta z + \ln(t_1 t_2)^2 + \ln[U'(f)/U(f)], \qquad (5)$$

where $I_s(f)$ is the intensity transmission coefficient. The terms α_s^I and α_w^I are the intensity attenuation coefficients of the sample and of water respectively. Henceforth, these superscripts will be dropped and any attenuation coefficients referred to in the text relate specifically to intensity.

Contributions to the total loss due to attenuative propagation in the sample and interfacial acoustic impedance mismatch are evident in equation 5. The remaining term, $\ln[U'(f)/U(f)]$ is the least tractable. It is important to recognise the origin of the term, albeit in a rather qualitative way, in order that its contribution to the total measured signal loss be minimised. It represents the relative change in the pressure distribution at a receiver of spatially finite extent invoked by the sample placement in the field. For a homogeneous material (where it will be assumed no scattering occurs) the quantity will be dependent on refraction if there is a sample to water velocity mismatch but will be accentuated by, (1) sample interfaces which may not be planar and parallel, and (2) any sample misalignment in the experimental set-up. The latter may be minimised by careful experimental procedure, whilst the former depends on sample preparation.

For measurements on castor oil and also for tissue-mimicking materials in general the velocities of propagation, c, are close to that of water. For example, for castor oil[8] at 20°C, c = 1505.7 ms⁻¹, whilst for degassed-deionised water at the same temperature c = 1482.4 ms⁻¹. In this case the uncertainty due to refraction should be negligible. Consequently equation 5 becomes

$$\ln[I(f)] = -(\alpha_s - \alpha_w)\Delta z + \ln(t_1 t_2)^2 \qquad (6)$$

Equation 6 provides the basis of the measurement procedure used in this study. Samples of different path length, Δz, were introduced at nominally identical positions along the acoustic axis and their transmission characteristics recorded.

11.3 Experimental details

11.3.1 Standard liquid reference cells

The requirement for a range of test liquid acoustic path lengths led to the manufacture of standard liquid reference cells. These are shown in *figure 11.2,* and consist of stainless steel chambers of outside diameter 80 mm and aperture 50 mm. Each face was machined to accept a Viton "o"-ring and polycarbonate face-plate.

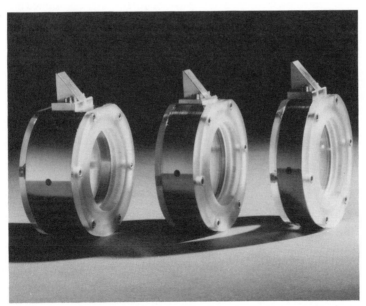

Figure 11.2   The standard liquid reference cells of thickness 5, 10 and 20 mm.

When the face-plate is clamped to the body it tensions the thin membrane material. The window material chosen for this particular application was Mylar (polyethylene terephthalate film) of thickness 9 μm because it has high strength and durability and has an acoustic impedance close to that of water. The cells were manufactured with nominal geometrical path lengths of 5, 10 and 20 mm. The specified manufacturing tolerance was ± 0.05 mm but in reality deformation due to tensioning and hydrostatic pressure would be expected to provide the greatest contribution to thickness uncertainties. Filler holes were provided in the chamber sides and all cells were syringe-filled with BDH laboratory Reagent grade castor oil at room temperature.

11.3.2 The measurement rig

The rig assembly was designed as a general purpose material characterisation facility for the measurement of attenuation, velocity, and scattering. The hardware, shown in *figure 11.3*, consists of three assembly carriages mounted on a pair of parallel cylindrical rails. Each carriage may be translated smoothly along the acoustic axis (z-direction) and clamped rigidly and reproducibly at any appropriate position. The transducer, test sample holder and receiver are suspended from assemblies mounted onto these carriages. Translations in the x, y and z directions are provided by standard optical bench micropositioning equipment. All three may be rotated about the x and y axes. Although conceived as a versatile measurement system, the rig was designed more specifically for the measurement of attenuation and velocity by the substitution method and some of

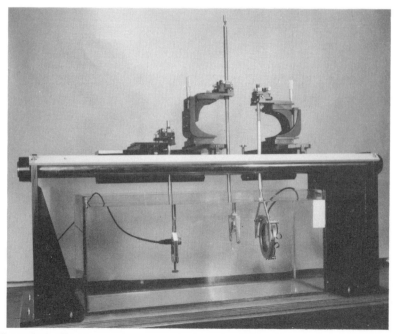

Figure 11.3 The materials characterisation measurement rig.

its features reflect this. The test sample may be swung out of the acoustic beam and replaced with an estimated precision of ± 0.1 mm. Provision has also been made to swing the sample out of the test tank completely, replace it with a second standard reference cell and return the new cell to a nominally identical position (to within, it is estimated, 0.2 mm).

11.3.3 Experimental

(a) System configuration

Details of the electrical drive and detection systems as well as the overall rig experimental configuration are shown in *figure 11.4*. The interrogating transducers used in this investigation were plane-piston Panametrics transducers of frequencies 2.25, 3.5, 5.0, 7.5 and 10.0 MHz, driven by the amplified gated output of a frequency generator. Using variable pulse-length tone-bursts, discrete frequency measurements were made at the nominal transducer centre frequencies.

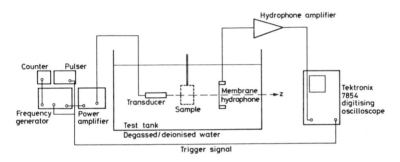

Figure 11.4 The experimental configuration used during this study.

The receivers used were PVDF hydrophones of the membrane type. These devices have become well established in ultrasonic field characterisation and will not be described here. Details of their performance characteristics are given by Preston *et al*. Of importance in the context of the present study is their wide bandwidth (25 MHz for the particular device used). Consequently, any harmonics of the fundamental transducer excitation frequency generated by nonlinear propagation through the water medium or the sample itself may be detected. The degassed-deionised water was maintained at the required measurement temperature by a FH15 Grant circulatory heater pump system and two stainless steel heat exchange coils (not shown in *figure 11.3*) situated in the test tank. The water temperature was measured with an uncertainty of ± 0.1°C.

The two sets of sample cells were stored in the test tank throughout the measurement period to aid thermal equilibration.

The hydrophone signal was amplified and displayed on a Tektronix 7854 waveform processing oscilloscope. The digitising capacity of this instrument permits the determination of the required signal averaged pulse parameters.

(b)   Measurement procedure

Alignment of the hydrophone on the acoustic axis of the test transducer was performed in the usual way. The liquid reference cell was placed in the transducer far-field, with typical source-sample separations of 1.3 to 1.8 near-field distances, and centred on the acoustic axis. The provision of two orthogonal rotational axes permitted the parallel alignment of the Mylar windows with the transducer and hydrophone faces. The hydrophone was placed just beyond the sample position, at 1.5 to 2.0 near-field distances. The sample cell was swung out of the acoustic beam for the reference measurement in water.

The transducer drive-voltage was maintained at a level such that there was no observed distortion of the received sinusoidal signal due to nonlinear propagation through the water or the sample. The length of the applied electrical drive tone-burst had to satisfy two criteria. Firstly, it had to be of sufficient duration to provide a region in the received waveform of constant amplitude. Secondly, to avoid reverberation effects, the pulse length had to be less than the sample interface-to-interface transit time. This second requirement is a problem at low frequencies although in reality the reflection coefficient of the water/Mylar/castor oil interface is small (less than 3 per cent at 2.25 MHz). Tone-bursts of 8 to 20 cycles were used throughout this study.

An isolated flat portion of the received waveform was digitised and the signal averaged peak-to-peak voltage determined. The sample cell was returned to its aligned on-axis position and the digitisation procedure repeated over the equivalent portion of the attenuated time-shifted waveform. The test sample was swung out of the tank, replaced with a new cell, and returned to the original location where the measurement procedure was repeated.

11.4   Results

The results obtained, represented by the full circles, are shown in *figure 11.5* alongside data obtained by two previous studies[5, 10]. The error bars shown represent the random uncertainties expressed at the 95 per cent confidence level. During the study, the temperature was maintained nominally at 30°C although excursions of up to ± 0.3°C were recorded for some measurements.

11.5   Discussion

11.5.1   Comparison with previous data

Measurements of the attenuation coefficient of castor oil were obtained by Dunn and Breyer[10] using a thermocouple technique over the frequency range 1–100 MHz. Harris *et al*[5] obtained their results using a broadband transmission substitution technique and signal-to-noise problems restricted their measurement frequency range to 1–5 MHz. Consequently the data of *figure 11.5* have been extrapolated over the full frequency range used for the present study. A detailed comparison of the three data sets is provided in *table 11.1*. With the exception of the 3.5 MHz measurement, the results of the present study are in agreement with both sets of data within the limits of the random uncertainty. However, the attenuation coefficients derived from the present work are between 1.5 per cent and 3.0 per cent higher over the frequency range studied. The source and significance of this apparent systematic difference requires further investigation.

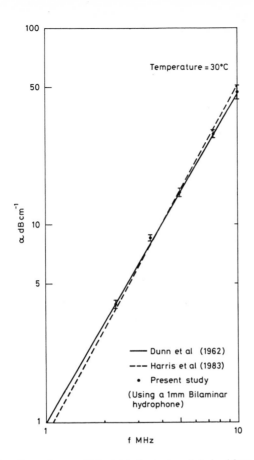

Figure 11.5 The attenuation coefficient data for castor oil derived from the present study displayed with the results of other two studies[5, 10].

Table 11.1 Tabulated intercomparison of values of the attenuation coefficient (α) for castor oil derived from the present measurements with the results of two previous studies[5, 10].

f (MHz)	α (dB cm^{-1})			Random uncertainty (95% confidence level)
	Harris *et al*[5]	Dunn and Breyer[10]	Present study	
2.25	3.70	3.84	3.93	4.6%
3.5	8.08	8.00	8.57	3.1%
5.0	15.20	14.46	14.77	6.1%
7.5	31.14	28.40	28.87	4.8%
10.0	51.80	45.70	47.14	8.3%

11.5.2 Uncertainties

Temperature. The present study has demonstrated the need for good control and accurate measurement of temperature in studies of this kind. The attenuation coefficient of castor oil is very temperature dependent; typically at 30°C and 2.25 MHz its value varies by 0.2 dB cm^{-1} per °C. Uncertainties in temperature due to spatial variations and thermal drift of ± 0.3°C would contribute ± 1.5 per cent to the random uncertainty of the measured attenuation coefficients in the frequency range 2.25–10.00 MHz.

Castor oil variations. The differing purity grades of castor oil available could exhibit different attenuation characteristics, but this uncertainty is impossible to quantify.

Transducer stability. This could introduce a random uncertainty of ± 3–4 per cent, depending on the characteristics of the test transducer.

Receiving system linearity. In the case of nominally 10 mm cell, the dynamic range of typical sample cell-water reference measurements varied from 2 dB at 2.25 MHz to 25 dB at 10.0 MHz. In this range, linearity deviations for both the hydrophone and hydrophone amplifier are negligible. However, a systematic uncertainty of ± 2 per cent may be attributed to nonlinearity in the oscilloscope plug-in amplifier.

Signal-to-noise ratio. This was a limitation at the higher measurement frequencies where it was not possible to obtain stable triggering of the received signal, although improvements in the signal-to-noise ratios could be obtained by using hydrophones of larger active element diameter. However, attenuation measurements on inhomogeneous media such as the tissue-mimicking materials may be subject to phase-cancellation effects[11] which could provide an additional source of uncertainty when using large receivers.

Refraction. During this work there was no observed dependence of the sample cell transmission coefficient on the sample cell to hydrophone separation, indicating that any refraction effects were smaller than the random uncertainties of the measurement. Harris *et al*[5] have estimated the effect to be less than one per cent. Refraction due to non-planar wavefronts and curved water-sample interfaces will result in a systematic uncertainty in the measured transmission coefficient that varies from cell to cell and with frequency. If beam-spreading effects are important then, for any particular cell, this will contribute to the random uncertainty due to sample alignment repeatability. This contribution will be particularly significant at high frequencies due to the directional response of the hydrophone. The indications are that the contributions that these effects make to the measured attenuation coefficients are small. This requires corroboration from further experimental and theoretical studies.

Nonlinear propagation. If the acoustic pressures used for the measurements are of a sufficiently high level, then nonlinear propagation of the ultrasound from source to sample or to the hydrophone will become important. The phenomenon is characterised by a progressive distortion of the initially sinusoidal waveform along the acoustic axis[12]. In a frequency domain representation, this distortion is accompanied by the generation of higher frequency harmonics of the drive transducer fundamental. The result is a non-monochromatic interrogating waveform and measured sample attenuation coefficients that are overestimates of the low amplitude discrete frequency values. The importance of this contribution in attenuation characterisation is currently being studied.

Sample cell thickness uncertainties. The random uncertainties were ± 1 per cent (expressed at the 95 per cent confidence level) for the optical determination of cell thickness. This would contribute $\pm$ 2 per cent to the attenuation coefficient random measurement uncertainty.

11.6 Summary

The early stages of a program designed to establish techniques for the characterisation of the acoustical properties of tissue-mimicking materials have been described. Attenuation measurements made on castor oil have been compared with two previous studies and good agreement has been demonstrated. Several sources of systematic and random uncertainty have been identified.

References

1 EGGLETON R C and WHITCOMB J A 1979 Tissue simulators for diagnostic ultrasound, in *Ultrasonic Tissue Characterisation II*, M Linzer ed, National Bureau of Standards Special Publn 525 (US Government Printing Office, Washington DC)
2 ZAGZEBSKI J A and MADSEN E L 1980 Ultrasonic Phantoms *IEEE Transactions on Nuclear Science* NS-27 1176-1182
3 BUSH N L and HILL C R 1983 Gelatine-alginate complex gel: a new acoustically tissue-equivalent material *Ultrasound in Medicine and Biology* 9 479-484
4 MADSEN E L, ZAGZEBSKI R A, BANJAVIC R A *et al* 1978 Tissue-mimicking materials for ultrasound phantoms *Medical Physics* 5 391-394
5 HARRIS R R, HERMAN B A *et al* 1983 *1983 Ultrasonics Symposium* 778-781
6 MADSEN E L, ZAGZEBSKI J A and FRANK G R 1982 Oil-in-gelatin dispersions for use as ultrasonically Tissue-mimicking materials *Ultrasound in Medicine and Biology* 8 277-287
7 DUNN F, EDMONDS P D and FRY W J 1969 in *Biological Engineering* (Edited by Schwan H P) p. 214 (McGraw-Hill, New York)
8 KAYE G W C and LABY T H in *Tables of Physical and Chemical constants* fourteenth edition (Longman, London)
9 PRESTON R C, BACON D R, LIVETT A J and RAJENDRAN K 1983 PVDF membrane hydrophone performance properties and their relevance to the measurement of the acoustic output of medical ultrasonic equipment *J Phys E: Sci Instrum* 16 786-796
10 DUNN F and BREYER J E 1962 Generation and detection of ultra-high-frequency sounds in liquids *J Acoust Soc Amer* 34 775-778
11 MARCUS P W and CARSTENSEN E L 1975 Problems with absorption measurements of inhomogeneous solids *J Acoust Soc Amer* 58 1334-1335
12 BEYER R T and LETCHER S V 1969 *Physical Ultrasonics* pp 202-241 (Academic Press, New York)

CHAPTER 12

Test Objects for the Assessment of the Performance of Doppler Shift Flowmeters

K McCarty and D J Locke
Bioengineering Unit, University Hospital of Wales, Heath Park, Cardiff CF4 4XW

12.1 Introduction

For some time now Test Objects and Test Procedures have been available for the characterisation of ultrasonic imaging equipment[1]. The existing devices, developed on funds from the Welsh Office and the DHSS and known collectively as the Cardiff Test System, are capable of characterising the stationary performance of imaging systems. A logical progression of this work, again funded by the DHSS, has been to encompass movement related parameters by providing new and complementary Test Objects.

This paper describes the design and fabrication of the first of these new devices, namely a Test Object for the assessment of performance of Doppler Shift Flowmeters.

It is anticipated that when these devices are available it will be possible to test all aspects of the performance of external contact scanners employing ultrasound.

12.2 Design requirements

When producing any test system for assessment, calibration and routine quality assurance, one of the first considerations is which parameters should be measured. This is best decided by studying the method of operation of equipment to be tested.

In general, diagnostic ultrasonic flowmeters indicate the velocity of blood flowing in vessels by utilising the Doppler-shifted frequency spectrum of a sound wave reflected from the moving blood. In their simplest form they provide an audible output of frequency. Measurement of the frequency (or frequency spectrum) will, when combined with the angle of inclination of the probe to the vessel, give an estimate of flow velocity. The combination of flow velocity with the cross-sectional area of the vessel will in turn provide an estimate of volume flow. Since diagnosis may be influenced by the numerical values of these estimations, checks must be made of the accuracy of velocity, vessel angle, vessel cross-sectional area, and volume flow measurement facilities. Bearing in mind that before data can be processed, it must first be collected, it is obvious that in addition to checking the accuracy of the computational facilities of devices, other parameters such as sensitivity, bandwidth or velocity range, separation of flow direction, aliasing threshold, and range gate accuracy need to be checked if the aim is to thoroughly assess the equipment.

Behind this oversimplified summary lies a whole series of measurement problems caused by the variation and limitations of the different types of Doppler equipment. A full discussion of these points is not appropriate here and the reader is refered to other authors[2-4] for a comprehensive treatment. It is maintained however, that careful study leads to the conclusion that the best, and perhaps only, way to uniformly check all Doppler ultrasound flowmeters is to model the important features of the systemic arterial network and provide a variable and calibrated 'patient'. Only in this way can we be sure of the relevance of the results. This approach also allows the system under test to be considered as a Black Box thus avoiding pitfalls such as assuming the universal availability of equipment test points, or testing the equipment as a series of independent parts. The remainder of this paper concentrates on the design of the model and leaves further discussion of the measurement of parameters until another time.

Taking the human arterial system as the design prototype for a model to assess Doppler shift flowmeters, it can be seen that the test object must contain tubes of various diameters at different depths, ranging perhaps from 1.5 mm bore near to the surface to 40 mm bore at depth. These tubes must contain a suitable 'blood like' fluid and this fluid must be pumped through the tubes in a number of predefined flow patterns.

If sensitivity measurements are to be valid the tubes and surrounding background material should be made from Tissue Mimicking Materal (TMM).

These gross features are implemented in the current test object which is of simple construction and operation and yet allows a full range of performance tests.

12.3 Materials and method

The bulk background material in the Test Object box is a carbon powder in gelatin mix giving the same stable TMM as is used in other Cardiff Test System test objects. The scattering fluid that has been used to date is a blood product consisting of a suspension of erythrocytes (red blood cells) preserved in gluteraldehyde. This material is easily prepared in a biochemical laboratory and has the advantage of being acoustically close to blood yet stable over many months.

Many materials have been considered for the tubing to stimulate arterial vessels, latex rubber being the present compromise. With regard to propagation velocity, dynamic properties, availability in a range of sizes, and reproducibility, it is very good. Other materials such as irradiated polyolefin tubing (heat shrink tubing)[5] and drinking straws have been considered, (see Results). The current prototype contains several latex tubes of different diameter and bore set at an angle of 30° to a scanning window which is specifically designed to allow visualisation of the tubes at almost zero depth. The connections to the tubing are external to the Test Object and can be connected in any order or flow direction required. In the present system they are connected 'radiator style' in order of decreasing tube diameter.

Versatility in the pumping of the scattering fluid has been achieved by having separate parallel generation of pulsatile and non-pulsatile flow components that can be summed to provide a composite waveform. Non-pulsatile flow is provided by a centrifugal pump which is more suitable for use in a closed system and produces less pulsation than for instance a gear pump. Degradation of the scattering particles, for example due to mechanical abrasion within the pump, must also be considered. Here again the centrifugal pump is best, having minimal effect on the fluid-suspended particles. The pumping head is magnetically coupled to the motor so as to prevent the introduction of air. The pulsatile component is provided by a peristaltic pump with a specially modified pump head. Many suitable waveforms can be reproduced. If very large pulsed volume flows are

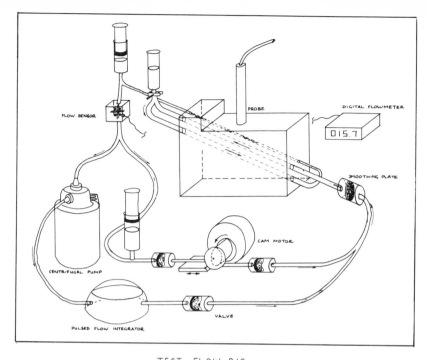

Figure 12.1   Schematic diagram of Test System layout.

required the two pumps can be connected in series. In this case the rollers of the cam act like valves controlling the head of fluid backed up by the continuous flow of the centrifugal pump.

Dampers at various points in the system introduce compliance (proportional to the volume of air in the closed chamber). This compliance is similar to that found in the arterial net. Compliance is a function analogous to the reciprocal of Youngs Modulus for the whole artery, but takes into account the dynamic and visco-elastic features of the artery. This compliance is known to vary in the clinical situation, for example in disease and old age. The dampers and latex tubing employed simulate this important parameter[6–8].

If unnecessary lengths of tubing are to be avoided laminar flow must be established soon after perturbing irregularities such as tube junctions. This is possible by the introduction of a suitable screen, for instance an 80 mesh filter[9].

As the system is a multi-pump configuration it cannot rely on a calibrated pump to indicate the volume flowing. An electro-mechanical flow sensor is incorporated.

The flow sensor in the current system is a Pelton wheel arrangement with four permanent magnets located at 90° intervals on the wheel. A Hall effect switch contained in the stationary housing is activated by each passing magnet. The rotational velocity of the wheel (determined by calculating the pulse rate from the

96

switch) is proportional to the total volume flow rate. Other types of flow sensors are being considered for improved response, (see Results).

The present system has a number of valves to limit the flow to one direction. They are necessary because of limitations of the present flow sensor. It can measure flow in either direction but as it gives out the same pulses irrespective of flow direction it will not reliably measure bi-directional flow, i.e. there is an over-estimation of the flow in any one direction.

The valves were specially designed to fulfil this relatively low pressure application as no suitable commercially available device could be found. They are a simple flap of thin material which blocks off flow through the support plate during negative flow.

The flow integrator is another air filled damper designed to remove any pulsatility from the continuous flow side of the system.

12.4 Results

With reference to tubing it is quite difficult to get an accurate measure of attenuation from the thin samples obtained by simply splitting open a thin walled tube. The relative attenuation is however quite easily assessed by immersing the tubes in TMM and scanning them with high frequency ultrasound (*figure 12.2*).

The latex tubing has a wall thickness of 1.5 mm and appears to reduce the beam by about 15 dB at 10 MHz. Therefore its attenuation is approximately 5 dB cm^{-1} MHz^{-1}.

A material proposed by McDicken[5] which looks interesting from the point of view of versatility of size and shape, and is thin walled, is irradiated polyolefin tubing. Unfortunately, it too is quite attenuating and this, together with its high rigidity and the unknown reproducibility of the material, makes it rather inappropriate for use as a substitute vessel in a test object. It may however be suitable for a number of geometric type tests such as range gate accuracy where thin rigid tubes are required.

Possibly a better option for the thin walled tube is the plastic drinking straw. Although here too there are uncertainties about the reproducibility of the material, it appears so transparent to ultrasound that minor batch to batch variation should not cause any serious problems. At present the drinking straw is being subjected to long term test to see if it is affected by the chemicals in the TMM, with a view to using it as one component of the Test Object.

This basic form has proved quite satisfactory with all the equipment tested except one high frequency transducer with an offset Doppler. The combination of low penetration, the flat-faced non rotatable transducer, the offset Doppler transducer, the limited range of acceptable probe to vessel angles and the critical angle at the tube-background interface, combine to prevent the velocity or volume flow computational facilities of the scanner being used. It is possible to get good waveforms but not at angles of inclination that the scanner will accept for computation. The production test object will therefore probably have some of the tubes set at a different angle to the window.

The standard peristaltic pump produces a long, slow, inflexible push. By changing the concave tube holder for a convex one with variable separation between the roller and the base, short sharp pulses of varying amplitude can be produced. By also changing the single roller to a very flexible multi-roller arrangement, giving essentially a cam, a wide range of pulse shapes can be obtained (*figure 12.3*).

97

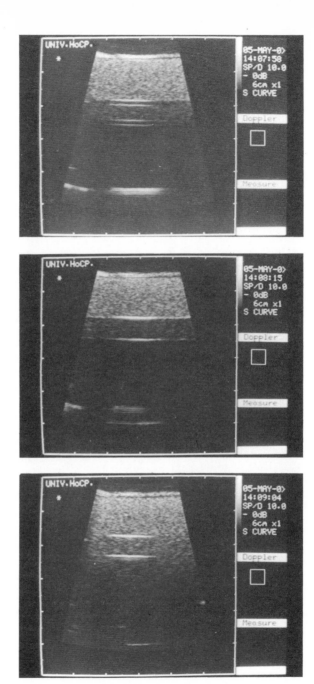

Figure 12.2 Scans of tubing embedded in TMM (a) Latex rubber, (b) Irradiated polyolefin, (c) Drinking straw.

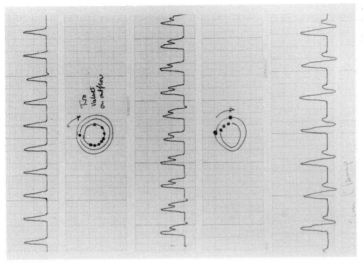

Figure 12.4 Maximum frequency waveforms produced in rig from two different cam configurations. The last waveform shows the effect on the dual pulse of removing the damping associated with the pump (see text).

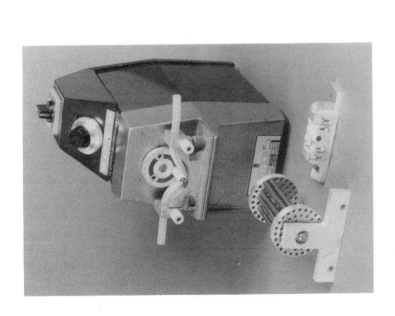

Figure 12.3 Commercial peristaltic pump together with the specially produced variable cam roller.

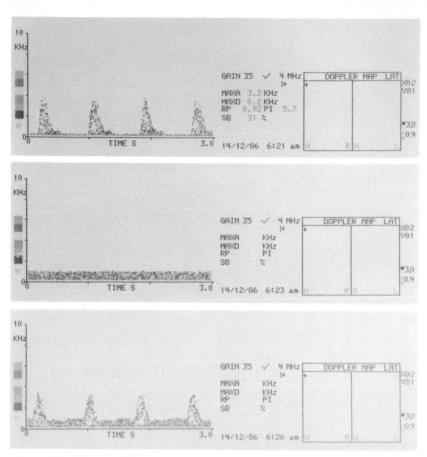

Figure 12.5 Doppler shift spectra of the output from the separate pulsed and continuous pumps and the result of combining the two.

A single roller gives a single pulse. Two rollers give a double pulse with the interval between them being controllable (bearing in mind the natural dynamics of the pipes) in terms of duration and flow rate. At present the system uses a commercial peristaltic pump for convenience. In the production model a more versatile stepper motor will be used which could for instance be made to reverse for a short part of its cycle and give a controllable reverse component. However this is not strictly necessary since negative flow can be turned on and off at will by controlling the compliance of the system. For instance, without a damper immediately before the cam there is a kind of suck-back after the roller disengages the pipe giving a negative flow component. With a damper in circuit there is sufficient pressure to provide a continuous forward flow when the roller disengages. At present the centrifugal pump produces a variable, but time independent, flow rate. By using an intelligent controller it is possible to vary the pump rate within each 'heart cycle' to produce complex simulations of clinical flow patterns.

100

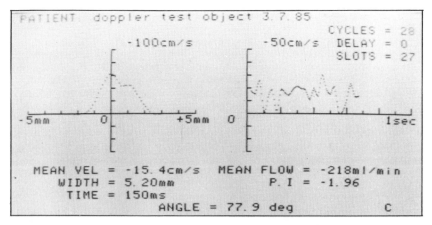

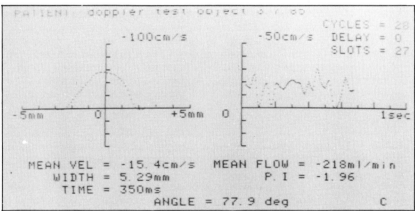

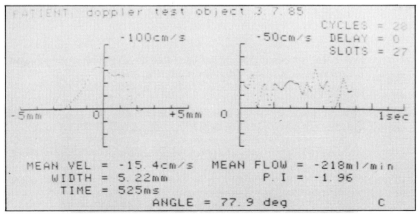

Figure 12.6 Flow profiles (measured with a multi-gated flowmeter) within the simulated vessel showing the approximation to parabolic flow during the cycle.

In order to check the computational capability of scanners it is important that the flow is laminar and the profile across the tube is known. Spectral analysis on many scanners indicates that the profile is probably parabolic.

This has been confirmed with a multi-gated flow mapper which showed that the profile is approximately parabolic at all times. Also, measurements of volume flow made on the flow mapper agree with the known flow through the test object to within 10 per cent, again indicating that the flow profile is acceptable (*figure 12.6*).

The flow sensor device[10] was quite accurate for non-pulsatile flow and for pulsatile flow up to about 100 pulses per second (pps). Beyond this rate the momentum of the relatively heavy magnets caused the paddle wheel to carry on spinning after the pulse had passed. This behaviour was quite easily seen in the impulse responses of the device[11, 12]. It has not yet been established whether in this region the flow sensor is acting as a pump and merely prolonging the pulse without inducing an error, or whether it is spinning in the fluid without pumping and hence giving a spurious reading of volume flow (*figure 12.7*).

The fast rise time of the impulse response indicates that there is very little chance of it spinning without pumping and that therefore it is suitable for relatively high volume uni-directional pulsed flow, but this has still to be confirmed.

Other flow sensors with better dynamic response exist and these are being investigated. One such device has an optical rotation detector[13] instead of magnets and the better dynamics afforded by a lighter paddle are reflected in its impulse response. This is estimated to be good for pulse rates above 200 pps. However since its optical sensor will not work in an opaque fluid such as blood it cannot be used in the rig. If no suitable flow sensor can be found at an acceptable price then this device can be modified to both work with blood and indicate flow direction.

If it is desired to check the ability of a scanner to pick up plaque by spectral broadening, control of the Doppler shift spectrum in the rig is important. The similarity to a radial artery of the waveforms shown demonstrates that this is clearly possible (*figure 12.8*).

Here again the system behaved as expected with the bandwidth in systole greater than in diastole. The next step in this area will obviously be to introduce further controlled spectral broadening in a tube. Until now no attempt has been made to simulate any particular vessel flow profile, but this is clearly possible.

12.5 Summary

A versatile and well specified flow rig has been described. Before being put into production, however, a number of points need further study.

The suspension of preserved red cells used as a whole blood substitute is adequate for development work but needs to be replaced by a non biological material. Several published suggestions are under investigation. Adoption of an existing, widely accepted substitute is desirable since it greatly eases the problems of standardisation of results between centres. It has, however, been difficult to obtain specific scattering particles so the final nature of the fluid has not yet been specified.

The latex rubber tubing has limitations with respect to its being thick walled and fairly attenuating. Studies are continuing in order to find the optimum vessel-stimulating tubing with appropriate acoustic and compliant properties.

The Pelton wheel flow sensor is adequate for uni-directional low pulsed volumes but not for high volume bi-directional pulsed flow. An affordable sensor

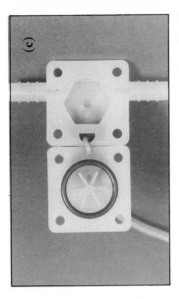

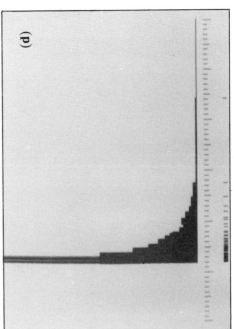

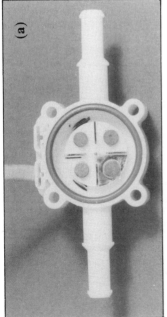

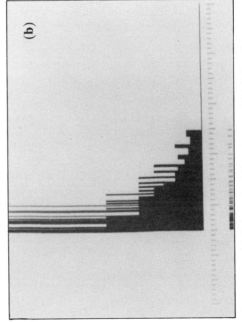

Figure 12.7 (a) Pelton wheel flow sensor and (b) its impulse response. (c) Optical rotation detector and (d) its impulse response. (N.B. The x-axis represents 6 seconds of time and the y-axis is relative rotational velocity).

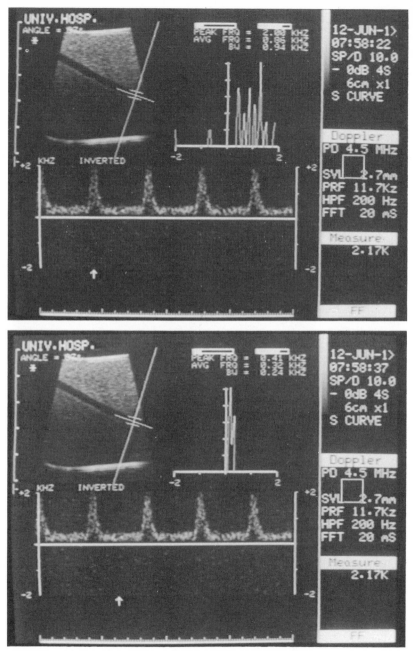

Figure 12.8 Duplex investigation of the working test rig. Note the desired spectral broadening during systole (a) compared to diastole (b).

with a superior dynamic response and bi-directional capability needs to be found or produced.

The production of complex flow waveforms using a combination of simple input flows has proved very successful and lends itself to quantification of the composite flow waveform. These flow waveforms/patterns are suitable for Doppler flowmeter volume flow calculation assessment. Further work needs to be done on the introduction of controlled spectral broadening.

12.6 Conclusions

It is anticipated that the above problems can be overcome in a relatively short time. The portable modular test object, in conjunction with comprehensive operator instructions, extends the Cardiff Test System to allow the assessment, calibration and quality assurance of diagnostic Doppler shift flowmeters.

The similarity of the test object to a portion of the systemic arterial net with associated compliance and acoustic properties ensures that the parameters are measured in a meaningful way. Amongst the parameters which can be assessed are:

Sensitivity
Receiver Bandwidth
Range Gate Accuracy
Pulsed Flow Velocity Calculation
Continuous Flow Velocity Calculation
Aliasing Threshold
Vessel Angle Measurement
Calculated Volume Flow
Separation of Flow Direction
Vessel Selectivity

In addition to the inbuilt versatility of the flow rig when assembled as described, the modular design and construction will lend itself to further adaption and experimentation by the user.

Acknowledgements

We would like to thank the Department of Health and Social Security for funding this work and Dr S Wilson of the Bioengineering Unit for much useful discussion.

References

1 .McCARTY K and STEWART W R 1985 'The Cardiff Test System', published by Diagnostic Sonar Ltd.
2 ATKINSON P and WOODCOCK J P 1982 *Doppler Ultrasound and its use in Clinical Measurement* (Academic Press, London)
3 EVANS D H 1986 Doppler ultrasound signals from blood flow, In: *Physics in Medical Ultrasound*, (Ed J A Evans) Chapter 15 (Institute of Physical Sciences in Medicine, London)
4 EVANS D H 1986 Can Duplex scanners really measure volumetric blood flow, In: *Physics in Medical Ultrasound* (Ed J A Evans) Chapter 19 (Institute of Physical Sciences in Medicine, London)

5   McDICKEN W N Design of test flow rig; Abstract from Quality Control in Medical Ultrasound meeting 24th October 1984, British Institute of Radiology

6   GUYTON C 1976 *Textbook of Medical Physiology* 5th edition (W B Saunders)

7   LIPPOLD D C J and WINTON F R 1979 *Human Physiology* 7th edition (Churchill Livingstone)

8   APERIA A 1940 Haemodynamic Studies *Skand Arch f Physiol* **83** Supplement 16

9   PERRY R H and CHILTON C H 1973 *Chemical Engineers Handbook* 5th Edition (McGraw-Hill)

10 R S Liquid flow sensors (R S Components Ltd, P O Box 99, Corby, Northants NN17 9RS)

11 JEPSON P and BEAN P G 1969 Effect of upstream velocity profiles on turbine flowmeter registration *J Mech Engng Sci* **11** 503–10

12 SCOTT R W W 1971 *Turbine Flowmeters Purchasing Directory for Process Industries* (Morgan Grampian Books, West Wickham, Kent)

13 FARNELL Precision flow sensor (Farnell Electronic Components Ltd, Canal Road, Leeds LS12 2TU)

CHAPTER 13

Geometric Distortion in Quality Control Images from Sector Scanners

R Price
Medical Physics Department, The General Infirmary, Leeds LS1 3EX

13.1 Introduction

The introduction in 1984 of the Cardiff system of test objects has led to the possibility of a standard series of measurements being made on ultrasound equipment throughout the country. However, if the full benefits of universal quality assurance testing are to be realised, care must be exercised in the acquisition and interpretation of results.

In Leeds Western District routine measurements on ultrasound scanners have already proved valuable in the demonstration of previously intractable problems. In particular, geometric distortion present in the image on one sector scanner has been identified and eliminated. In the process it was noted that all sector scanners tested exhibited some degree of distortion (*figure 13.1*), and it was in the interests of clarifying this issue that the following calculations were performed.

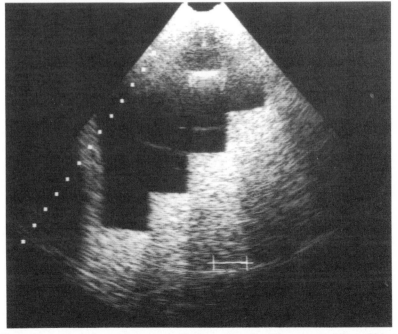

Figure 13.1 Typical sector scanner display using Cardiff grey-scale Test Object. Geometrical distortion is particularly evident near the edges of the sector.

107

13.2 Procedure

The Interpretation Notes, contained in part C of the manual for the Cardiff System, include curves showing how the parallel displacement of an ultrasound beam passing through the scanning window of a test object varies with incident angle. These have been generated by computing values for a plate (i.e. the window) rotated in a single medium. Problems arise when there are different media on either side of the plate, as for example when ordinary scanning jelly is used as a coupling medium. In such circumstances two other effects which alter the imaged position of points in the test object are introduced:

1. The beam assumes a completely new direction, the angle being that which would be given by refraction between the coupling medium and the tissue mimicking gel. This produces an error in imaged point position which is both depth and angle dependent.
2. The distance along the beam line, measured by the time delay between pulse transmission and echo reception, will not correspond to the true distance from transducer to imaged point. This error varies with scan angle due to varying path lengths in the curved wedge of couplant between the surface of the transducer and the test object scanning window.

It is relatively easy to calculate, by applying elementary optical formulae, the true position of a point whose apparent (i.e. imaged) position is known.

Let us consider the point I (*figure 13.2*), whose coordinates are r, θ, the origin being at the centre of rotation of the transducer. Point C is imaged as if it were at point I.

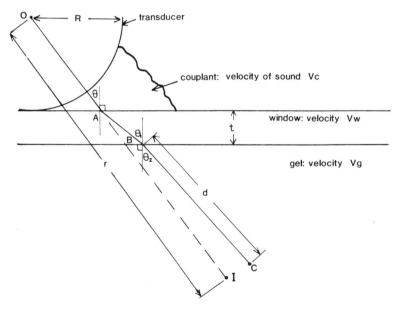

Figure 13.2 Diagram showing optical path for waves passing through the top of a Test Object using coupling gel.

108

From Snell's law $\quad \theta_1 = \arcsin\left(\dfrac{Vw}{Vc}.\sin\theta\right)$

and $\quad \theta_2 = \arcsin\left(\dfrac{Vg}{Vw}.\sin\theta_1\right)$

The length of path OA is $R/\cos\theta$, the cartesian coordinates of point A being $R.\tan\theta, -R$. Point B is at $t.\tan\theta_1, -t$ relative to A.

Path BC uses the rest of the measured time interval, say T_1. The total time interval, measured from the transducer surface, is

$$T = \frac{r-R}{Vg}$$

as the velocity of sound in the test object gel is designed to be the same as that in tissue, for which the scanner is calibrated.

The time used on path BC may be estimated by subtracting the known times used in the couplant and the window from the known total time, i.e.

$$T_1 = T - \frac{R}{Vc}\left(\frac{1}{\cos\theta} - 1\right) - \frac{t}{Vw.\cos\theta}$$

and the distance travelled in the test object gel is

$$d = T_1.Vg$$

Therefore $X = R.\tan\theta + t.\tan\theta_1 + d.\sin\theta_2$

and $\qquad Y = -R - t - d.\cos\theta_2$

It is probably more useful to calculate the imaged position of a point given the true position. In this case there is no analytical solution as θ, the angle at which the beam leaves the transducer, is not known. An iterative method was adopted as follows.

1. Assume that θ is the same as the angle between the normal from the centre of the transducer and the line joining the centre of the transducer to the object.
2. Calculate the x-coordinate of the image from
   $$X1 = R.\tan\theta + t.\tan\theta_1 + (Y-R-t).\tan\theta_2$$
3. Calculate a better approximation to θ
4. Calculate Y1, the y-coordinate of the image
5. If the correction was significant return to step 2, otherwise exit.

This was implemented in BBC Basic as a procedure, which was used in two main ways. The first was the calculation of tables of expected errors in image position for a range of transducer radii, couplant sound velocities, and X and Y positions. The other was in the plotting of the expected image positions of points in the test objects to provide a visual demonstration that the kind of distortion originally observed was at least partly due to these refraction effects.

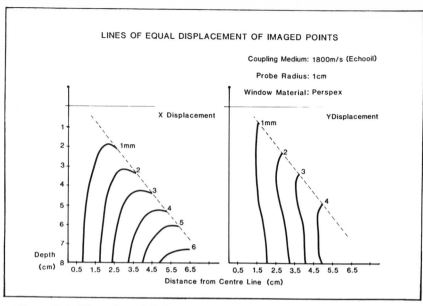

Figure 13.3 Lines of equal displacement of imaged points using echo oil as the coupling medium.

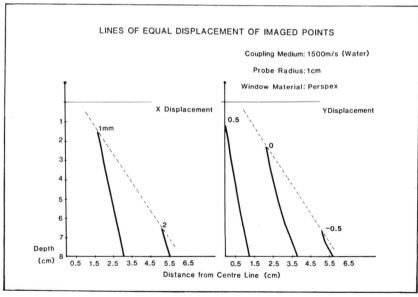

Figure 13.4 Lines of equal displacement of imaged points using water as the coupling medium.

110

13.3 Results

The tables of expected errors are cumbersome, containing thousands of entries, and are not easy to interpret. They do, however, provide useful corrections for measurements taken under less than ideal conditions.

To appreciate the magnitude of the problem likely to be encountered when using any given couplant it is helpful to present the data from the tables in a more readily assimilated form. The most convenient presentation was found to be a series of lines of equal error in image position, plotted against object position in the scan plane. X and Y errors were shown separately, and such pairs of charts were produced for different couplants, transducer radii, and window materials (*figures 13.3 and 13.4*). The errors were seen to be insensitive to changes in transducer radius and window material, only the velocity of sound in the couplant having any significant effect on the magnitude of the displacement.

The plots of imaged position of points in the test object demonstrated distortion markedly similar to that found on scanning the test objects with ordinary scanning oil as a couplant (*figure 13.5*). Distortion was minimal if a coupling medium with a velocity of sound similar to that of water was assumed.

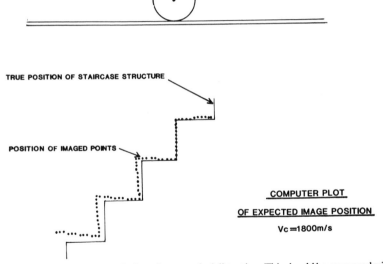

Figure 13.5   Computer prediction of geometrical distortion. This should be compared with *figure 13.1*.

13.4 Discussion

It is clear from the iso-displacement curves that significant distortion of the image occurs when the test objects are scanned through a couplant in which the velocity of sound differs from that in the test object filling. In particular, the scanning media to be found in most ultrasound departments, in which the velocity of sound is of the order of 1800 ms^{-1}, introduce displacement of imaged points by up to 7 mm. This would make it useless to attempt to check lateral caliper

111

accuracy. Comparison of scans through such media with similar scans made through water confirms the coupling medium as the origin of the distortion. Clearly, water should always be used when testing sector scanners; the collapsible plastic bags of saline supplied for drips are easy to use for this purpose once they have been partially emptied.

It is obviously of some value to determine whether this effect is important in routine clinical scanning. In fact, the pressure applied to the transducer is normally sufficient to deform the skin giving direct, orthogonal contact between transducer and subject over most of the scan field. Errors in measurement are, therefore, only likely to be significant near the edges of the scan. In circumstances which do not allow the skin to be deformed in this way a wide-angle image can only be produced if a wedge of couplant is built up; caliper measurements should then be confined to the centre of the field.

The other circumstance in which errors may occur is when a standoff medium is used. The standoff acts as a wedge of couplant, and distortion is introduced unless the velocity of sound in the standoff is close to 1540 ms^{-1}. Unfortunately, while water bag standoffs are quite acceptable, the solid medium which is commonly available has a sound velocity of 1380 ms^{-1} so a degree of distortion and consequent caliper error will be introduced.

13.5 Conclusion

When making any measurements, whether for clinical or quality control purposes, one should be acutely aware of the physical processes involved. In the case of ultrasound sector scanners the application of simple optical principles has demonstrated that apparent poor geometric performance may be due to lack of care in the choice of couplant. There are also implications for the accuracy of caliper measurements in clinical scanning under certain conditions.

CHAPTER 14

Quality Control of Ultrasonic Scanners — A Scheme for Routine Assessment

M J Lunt*
Rotherham District General Hospital, Moorgate Road, Rotherham, South Yorkshire S60 2UD
J M Pelmore (*Leicester*), W I J Pryce (*Sheffield*) and R Richardson (*Nottingham*)

14.1 Introduction

The need for routine quality control checks has now been recognised, but there is little practical information available on the use of these tests. A group of physicists from the Trent Region has recommended a scheme for routine assessment of scanner performance and the scheme has been evaluated over an 18 month period.

Assessment schemes can have two main aims — either to compare the performances of different scanners or to detect changes in performance of individual scanners. The Trent scheme is intended to detect changes in performance and no attempt is made to measure parameters absolutely. This simplified the choice of parameters to be included.

It is important that any assessment scheme is applicable to a wide range of ultrasonic instruments, including static B scanners, linear array scanners, curved array sector scanners, mechanical sector scanners and phased array sector scanners. The Trent scheme is designed to be applicable to all these types, and this limited the choice of test object.

14.2 Choice of parameters

A report[1] published by the Hospital Physicists' Association in 1978 listed six parameters that could be measured (caliper accuracy, system sensitivity, registration accuracy, axial resolution, dynamic range and output power or intensity) and emphasised that only three of these (caliper accuracy, system sensitivity and dynamic range) were relatively easy to measure.

Because the Trent scheme is designed to detect changes in equipment performance, it is only necessary to examine independent parameters and it is therefore possible to reduce the above list since changes in dynamic range, axial resolution and output intensity are all likely to affect system sensitivity. The Trent scheme therefore includes only three parameters: caliper accuracy, system sensitivity and registration accuracy.

14.3 Choice of test objects

Many test objects could have been used, including a delay line, a perspex block, an AIUM test object, a tissue-mimicking test object, and an ASIST pulse generator. All of these can be used to check caliper accuracy along the ultrasonic beam but only an AIUM test object and a tissue-mimicking test object can be used to check

Present address: Poole General Hospital, Dorset BH15 2JB

caliper accuracy when measuring across the beam direction of a sector scanner. Because it was felt important to devise a scheme using a single low cost test object, the AIUM device[2] was chosen as the cheapest object suitable for checking all three parameters on the full range of scanners. This is a fluid filled phantom with accurately positioned wires as echo generating targets. The fluid is a water/alcohol mixture in which the ultrasound velocity is 1540 ms^{-1} at room temperature. An additional reason for selecting the AIUM phantom was that the filling medium is stable. This is essential for sensitivity tests, and data on the long term stability of tissue-mimicking materials was not available when the scheme was devised.

14.4 Accuracy of measurement

The three parameters, caliper accuracy, system sensitivity and registration accuracy need to be assessed sufficiently precisely for changes to be detected before they become clinically significant. Calipers are used for fetal biparietal diameter measurements and it has been shown[3] that the operator inaccuracy is at least 1 per cent (one standard deviation). Ideally caliper calibration error should be less than about one third of this value.

Information on detectable changes of sensitivity is not readily available but a change of 3 dB is unlikely to be important clinically. Registration errors are

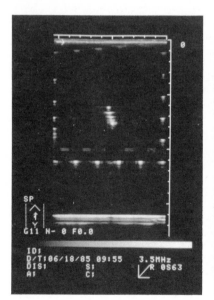 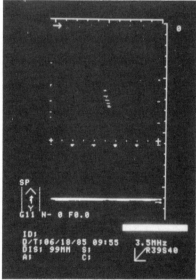

Figure 14.1 Grey scale image of the AIUM test object using a linear array scanner. The base of the test object can be seen as a horizontal line 16 cm deep — this can be used to check uniformity of sensitivity across the beam.

Figure 14.2 Bistable display of the same frozen image as *figure 14.1*. The reject level is given by the figures at the bottom right (Reject 39, Saturation 40). The calipers are positioned as nearly as possible over the maxima of the echoes.

important mainly in compound scanning and again there is a lack of information. However, an absolute measure of error can be made using the AIUM object, and an error of less than 5 mm at distances up to 15 cm is assumed to be acceptable.

14.5 Caliper accuracy — measurement procedure

Caliper accuracy is assessed by scanning the AIUM phantom and positioning calipers on the image both vertically (along the ultrasonic beam) and horizontally (across the beam) on echoes from wires 10 cm apart. For each test the controls are fixed in predetermined positions, chosen to make the two echoes approximately the same amplitude. The probe is moved until both echoes are at maximum amplitude and the display frozen (*figure 14.1*).

For measurements along the beam, the calipers are positioned either on the leading edges of the echoes or on the echo maxima. For measurements across the beam, they are positioned on the echo maxima. The position of the maximum can be accurately determined using the post-storage processing if this is available. By altering the relationship between stored echo amplitude and display brightness, a bistable display can usually be obtained. This has all echoes stored at or below a reject level displayed as black, and all above this level displayed as white. As the reject level is increased, the last part of the echo to disappear is the maximum. The calipers can then be placed over the maximum of each echo and the separation recorded (*figure 14.2*).

It is important to note that the calipers positioned across the beam on sector scanners do not always read 100 mm for a 100 mm wire separation. This is because of increased velocity and refraction in the plastic top of the test object and the coupling medium, as Mr Price has shown in the previous paper (Chapter 13). However, because it is only a change in reading that is significant, this problem is overcome. Inconsistencies in the results may be due to angling of the scanning plane, changes in test object temperature and incorrect caliper positioning. Angling of the plane is overcome by looking for maximum echo amplitude and incorrect caliper positioning is overcome by using the post-storage processing. Velocity of ultrasound in the water/alcohol mixture changes by about 0.1 per cent per °C so an absolute difference of only ± 3°C is acceptable. A phantom with an integral thermometer is recommended.

The main difficulty in caliper assessment is due to the quantisation of readings to the nearest millimetre in the majority of real time scanners. This prohibits accuracy better than 1 per cent and means that the target accuracy of 0.3 per cent cannot be achieved. However, a 1 per cent accuracy has been found acceptable for regular use.

14.6 System sensitivity — measurement procedure

System sensitivity is assessed by imaging a particular wire in the phantom and determining the maximum echo amplitude from that wire. It is important that the same wire is used and that the scanner controls are fixed in predetermined positions, chosen to give a convenient amplitude. The probe is placed on the phantom and the position adjusted to give maximum echo amplitude.

If post storage processing is available, it can be used to ensure an echo amplitude close to maximum. The processing is adjusted to give a bistable display as indicated above and the reject level set slightly below the anticipated maximum amplitude. As the probe is moved, a more sensitive indication of the maximum is

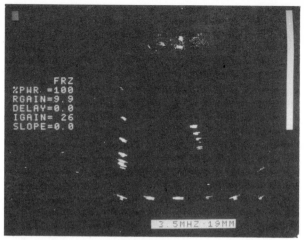

Figure 14.3 Bistable image of the AIUM test object using a mechanical sector scanner. The reject level has been adjusted to assist in finding the maximum echo amplitude. The second wire from the left on the bottom row is usually used for sensitivity checks.

achieved and the image can be frozen to store the maximum (*figure 14.3*). The actual amplitude is recorded by measuring the reject level required to obliterate the echo.

If post storage processing is not available, one of the controls affecting gain has to be adjusted until the echo just fails to appear on the real time image. This can be difficult to determine and it can also be difficult to record accurately the position of the control. However, in general these problems can be overcome without prolonging the procedure unduly and a reproducible result achieved.

The main inconsistencies in the results occur due to angling of the scanning plane, and it is important that the correct angle is obtained. Poor acoustic coupling can also cause echo reduction, and liberal use of coupling medium is essential, in particular when testing sector scanners.

This test only measures sensitivity at one position in the image, and for array scanners there could be faulty transducer elements causing local sensitivity reduction. Uniformity from a linear array can be checked by examining the reflection from the base of the phantom (see *figure 14.1*) or by moving the transducer and observing the image of a particular wire as it moves through the field. This latter method can also be used for sector scanners and the sensitivity of the test can be improved by setting the controls so that the echo is close to threshold before the test is performed. At present this test is only done qualitatively, but a more rigorous examination could be made if a fault were suspected.

14.7 Registration accuracy — measurement procedure

Registration accuracy is only applicable to static B scanners, and is assessed by imaging a particular wire in the phantom from several different directions. It is important that the same wire is used and that control settings are fixed with the

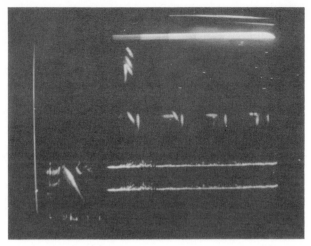

Figure 14.4 Grey scale magnified image of part of the phantom using a static B scanner. The wires have been scanned from different directions and each appears as a group of lines. Misregistration is given by the maximum separation of the centres of the lines from a given wire. The parallel horizontal lines at the bottom are 1 cm calipers used for scaling.

image at maximum magnification. The target is scanned from four directions, two horizontal, one vertical and one oblique. The image of the wire appears as 4 separate lines on the screen, which should all intersect at their centres. Misregistration is determined by measuring the maximum distance between the centres of a pair of lines (*figure 14.4*).

It is important that the scanning plane is not angled in relation to the phantom, and that temperature effects do not alter the velocity of ultrasound in the phantom.

14.8 Experience with the scheme

The scheme was assessed by using it regularly four times per year for 18 months on 3 different scanners (linear array, B scanner and mechanical sector). Results over the period indicate that the sensitivity can be measured to 1 dB using the post storage processing and that calipers can be assessed to the nearest millimetre.

Two definite performance changes were found during the test period. These were a sensitivity change in the linear array scanner following servicing and an incorrect caliper setting on the B scanner after servicing. In addition, the sensitivity of the sector scanner could not be assessed because of substantial drift in output intensity after switching on. The scheme has also been tried once with a convex linear scanner and assessment proved possible provided a liberal amount of coupling medium was used. Significant distortion of the test object image was observed due to increased horizontal separation of echoes distant from the probe (*figure 14.5*). Mr Price, in the previous paper, has shown this to be due to an increased ultrasonic velocity through the coupling medium.

117

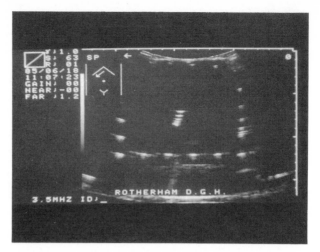

Figure 14.5 Grey scale image of the phantom using a convex linear scanner. The probe was coupled to the phantom using gel and this causes visible distortion of the image. The bottom wires registered 103 mm separation instead of the 100 mm true separation.

14.9 Conclusion

The Trent scheme has been designed to detect changes in equipment performance by examining caliper accuracy, system sensitivity and registration accuracy. It requires an AIUM test object, and the model with an integral thermometer is recommended.

The scheme has been used over an 18 month period on a variety of scanners and changes around 1 dB in sensitivity and 1 per cent in caliper accuracy are detectable. A measurement frequency of four times per year with additional checks after servicing has been found to be satisfactory.

References

1   HOSPITAL PHYSICISTS' ASSOCIATION 1978 *Methods of Monitoring Ultrasonic Scanning Equipment* — Topic Group Report 23 (Hospital Physicists' Association, 47 Belgrave Square, London SW1X 8QX)
2   AMERICAN INSTITUTE FOR ULTRASOUND IN MEDICINE 1974 *Standard 100 millimeter Test Object Manual* — Publication Number 331 (AIUM Publications, 4405 East-West Highway, Suite 504, Bethesda, Maryland, 20814, USA)
3   LUNT R M and CHARD T 1974 Reproducibility of measurement of fetal biparietal diameter by ultrasonic cephalometry *Journal of Obstetrics and Gynaecology of the British Commonwealth* **81** 682–685

CHAPTER 15

Doppler Ultrasound Signals from Blood Flow

D H Evans
Department of Medical Physics and Clinical Engineering, Leicester Royal Infirmary, Leicester LE1 5WW

15.1 Introduction

Ultrasonic waves which have been reflected or scattered from moving targets within the body will be shifted in frequency with respect to the transmitted waves due to the Doppler effect. This physical phenomenon forms the basis of the large number of Doppler 'velocimeters' now available. The method has the major advantage that it allows measurements to be made non-invasively from intact vessels under physiological conditions, without in any way interfering with the flow being measured. The technique is also thought to be entirely safe, provided efforts are made to keep the power levels used within reasonable limits. Satomura[1] is credited with describing the first successful use of an ultrasonic Doppler device to monitor blood flow, and since then a number of innovations have led to the modern, relatively sophisticated device, which can determine the direction of flow, calculate mean flow velocity, provide information about velocity distributions, and may allow the signals from a particular range of depths to be isolated and analysed. The basic Doppler principle is extremely simple, but its application to the measurement of blood flow is complicated by many additional factors, some of which will be discussed in this chapter.

Doppler devices may be either continuous wave (CW) or pulsed wave (PW). There are a number of fundamental differences between the two types of device, and each has its own merits.

15.2 Continuous wave Doppler

Continuous wave Doppler units transmit a continuous monochromatic ultrasound wave into the tissue which is thus reflected and back-scattered to some degree (until the attenuation along the path length effectively quenches the wave) from every 'target' which lies in the path of the beam. The ultrasound beam is manipulated so that only one vessel lies in its path and the best possible signal obtained, and the resulting Doppler shift signal is used to characterise or measure the flow within the vessel.

The Doppler shift frequency f_d produced by a blood cell moving through an infinitely wide ultrasound beam is given by the well known equation:

$$f_d = f_t - f_r = (2f_t v \cos \theta)/c \qquad (1)$$

where f_t and f_r are the transmitted and received ultrasound frequencies, v is the velocity of the target, c the velocity of sound in tissue, and θ the angle between the probe axis and the direction of travel of the cell. In reality the ultrasound beam cannot be treated as infinitely wide and in any blood flow measurement situation there are numerous targets in the ultrasound field with a range of velocities, and thus the Doppler shift signal contains not a single frequency, but rather a spectrum of frequencies which varies as the blood flow distribution changes from moment to moment. Since the Doppler shift frequency is proportional to velocity, and the power in any frequency band is proportional to the number of erythrocytes travelling with velocities which conduce frequencies in that band, the Doppler power spectrum would under 'ideal' conditions have the same shape as a velocity distribution plot for the flow in the vessel. In practice there are a number of other factors which influence the Doppler power spectrum and limit the accuracy with which the velocity distribution in the vessel can be determined.

15.2.1 Non-uniform insonation

Non-uniform insonation of the blood vessel can significantly change the shape of the Doppler power spectrum, and invalidate any conclusions which are drawn about the velocity distribution or mean velocity within a vessel. In general, narrow beams tend to emphasise the flow at the centre of the vessel at the expense of the relatively slow moving flow near to the walls. This leads to spectra with accentuated high frequencies and to an overestimation of mean velocity. Illustrations of the effect of non-uniform insonation on the shape of the power spectrum can be found in *reference 2,* whilst its effect on the determination of mean flow velocity is discussed in *reference 3.* The beam shapes of a number of commercial CW wave transducers (measured in water baths) have been published[4,5], but it was found in both of these studies that probes of the same type do not necessarily produce identical or even nearly identical field patterns, and that it is therefore necessary to make measurements on every probe that is to be used in an application where beam shape is critical.

15.2.2 Non-uniform target distribution

Scattering of ultrasound from blood is almost entirely due to the erythrocytes[6], but because of interference effects the intensity of the backscattered signal is proportional to the mean square fluctuations in the local cell concentration $<\Delta n^2>$, rather than the actual cell concentration itself[7]. In general ultrasound is equally scattered from the entire cross-section of a vessel, but it has been found that turbulence increases the amount of scattering that occurs[6]. Angelsen[7] has suggested that this is a result of local acceleration in the velocity field causing a separation between cells and plasma due to their different mass densities, and a consequent increases in $<\Delta n^2>$. The amount by which the scattering is increased is as yet undetermined, but it is a common observation that signals from turbulent jets are relatively strong. Velocity spectra recorded from highly turbulent flow must therefore be treated with caution.

15.2.3 Spectral broadening

Each target which passes through the ultrasound beam scatters a burst of ultrasound which has a zero-crossing frequency determined by equation 1. The frequency domain representation of such a burst is a spectrum with a relative width $(\Delta f_r/f_r)$ given approximately by the reciprocal of the number of oscillations in the burst (the exact relationship depends on the shape of the modulating function and the definition of spectral width), and centred on f_r. The relative spectral broadening in the RF signal results in a similar relative spectral broadening of the Doppler shift signal, and thus the Doppler shift from even a

120

single target has a finite bandwidth. It can be shown that the bandwidth to centre frequency ratio $\Delta f/f$ is given by:

$$\Delta f/f \simeq \lambda \tan \theta / 2w \qquad (2)$$

where λ is the wavelength of the ultrasound beam and w its width. Provided the ultrasound beam is much wider than λ (and this is a necessary condition if the beam is to be reasonably parallel) then this broadening will lead to only a slight smearing of the Doppler spectrum, and is of little consequence in practice.

15.2.4 Attenuation

Attenuation is higher in soft tissues than in blood and this reduces the relative sizes of echoes from the edge of the vessel and thus has the same effect as reducing the width of the ultrasound beam. This effect becomes greater as the angle θ decreases, and is more pronounced at higher frequencies thus exacerbating the effect of non-uniform insonation. Cobbold et al[8] have documented this effect for ultrasound beams with square and Gaussian shapes. Since the bandwidth to centre frequency ratio of the scattered ultrasound beam is small, frequency dependent attenuation effects can be ignored for CW Doppler.

15.2.5 Filtering

In addition to the Doppler shifted signal arising from blood flowing through the ultrasonic field, there is inevitably a component of the Doppler signal that arises from other moving structures such as the vessel wall. Fortunately most of these signals are of low frequency, but they may have amplitudes which are considerably greater than those from the blood. It is therefore necessary to incorporate a high-pass filter into the Doppler unit, and in addition to removing the unwanted clutter signal it will remove the signal returning from blood which has a low velocity. This leads to a distortion of the power spectrum and an overestimate of the mean velocity of flow. This effect has been discussed by Gerzberg and Meindl[9] and Gill[10].

15.2.6 Spectral analysis limitations

In order to extract the maximum amount of information from the Doppler signal it is necessary to transform it into the frequency domain. The performance of digital spectrum analysers is determined by the data sampling rate, the length of the data segments, and the way in which these segments are handled. The frequency resolution Δf_a is given by the reciprocal of the data collection time T_a, whilst the maximum frequency that can be correctly interpreted is given by half the sampling rate. Arterial Doppler signals cannot be considered stationary for periods of greater than about 10–20 ms, and it is therefore impossible to obtain a frequency resolution of better than about 50–100 Hz, even if the Doppler shift signal has a low frequency. The limited period of data collection also introduces a random inaccuracy into the determination of the amplitude of each frequency component. This is caused by the randomness of the relative positions of the individual blood cells and may be at least partially overcome by averaging spectral estimates either within the same beat (provided the total data segment used is less than or equal to the stationary period of the velocity), or over a number of beats. In the first case the reduction in amplitude variance is obtained only at the expense of frequency resolution.

15.3 Pulsed wave Doppler

A drawback of CW Doppler is that the Doppler shift signal may originate from anywhere along the ultrasound beam. This limitation may be overcome using a pulsed Doppler technique, which allows the Doppler signal to be range gated. An electronic gate is synchronised to the transmitter and is opened after a time delay T_d for a short period of time T_g. If the length of the transmitted pulse is T_p then only signals from targets with ranges of between (T_d-T_p) c/2 and (T_d+T_g) c/2 are detected. PW Units are used in either a long or short gate mode. In the former T_g is adjusted to be sufficiently large to receive echoes from the entire vessel and reject signals from outside the vessel; in the latter T_g is much shorter and signals from only a small part of the vessel are selected for analysis. The short gate technique is used mainly to study velocity profiles in detail and to detect localised turbulence. There are many similarities between the two PW techniques, and between these and CW techniques, but there are also a number of important differences which are discussed below.

15.3.1 Non-uniform insonation

Whilst CW transducers must necessarily use two crystals it is the usual practice in PW applications to use a single circular crystal for both transmitting and receiving. Hence the field shape produced by a PW unit differs from that from a CW unit both radially (due to crystal shape) and longitudinally (due to finite pulse length). The field produced by a circular vibrating piston excited in a CW mode (or by pulses containing several cycles) is well understood and is discussed in a number of text-books (e.g. *reference 11*), but the instantaneous field shapes resulting from short pulses can be quite complicated (see for example *reference 12*), and can usually only be calculated numerically. As with CW Doppler it is essential that the field from a long-gate Doppler unit is substantially uniform over the entire lumen of the vessel if the Doppler power spectrum is to be representative of the velocity distribution in the vessel, and so in addition to the gate being sufficiently broad to encompass the whole vessel, the ultrasound beam must also be sufficiently wide. Short-gate Doppler units do not insonate the vessel uniformly and would ideally reflect the velocity distribution of the erythrocytes in the small sample volume they interrogate. Unfortunately spectral broadening mechanisms become important in such instances (see next section) and considerable care must be taken with the interpretation of such spectra.

15.3.2 Spectral broadening

In CW applications spectral broadening is determined by the width of the ultrasound beam, in PW applications it is determined by the transmitted pulse length, and the bandwidth to centre frequency ratio $\Delta f/f$ is given simply by the reciprocal of the number of cycles in the transmitted burst. Considerable spectral broadening occurs where very short pulses are used, and it is thus difficult to distinguish between broadening caused by a true distribution of velocities in the sample and that due to the use of a short pulse. This is a fundamental limitation due to the finite wavelength of the ultrasound. The use of pulses with large bandwidths creates an additional problem in that as both scattering and attenuation are frequency dependent, the shape of a short pulse can be considerably distorted as it travels through the body and is scattered by the blood cells. *Figure 15.1* illustrates the changes in the normalised power spectrum of a pulse of ultrasound as it is attenuated on the way to the target, scattered from the

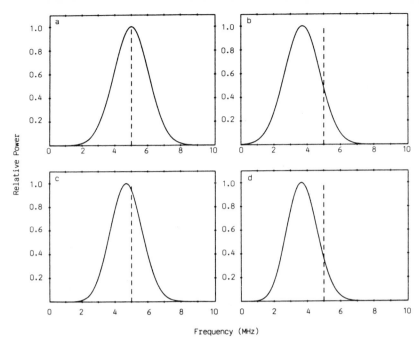

Figure 15.1 The effect of frequency dependent attenuation and scattering on the power spectrum of a short Gaussian pulse of bandwidth to centre frequency ratio of 0.5. The pulse has a centre frequency of 5 MHz, the target is located at 5 cm from the transducer, and the tissue has an attenuation of 1 dB/MHz/cm. (a) shows the power spectrum of the transmitted pulse, (b) the power spectrum following attenuation on the way to the target, (c) the scattered power spectrum, and (d) the power spectrum of the pulse arriving back at the transducer.

blood cell, and finally attenuated as it returns to the transducer. Newhouse *et al*[13] have shown that the ratio of the measured Doppler shift to correct Doppler shift f_d'/f_d for a sample volume in which all the scatterers have the same velocity is given by

$$f_d'/f_d = 0.5 \left(1 - \epsilon/\delta\right) + 0.5 \left[\left(1 - \epsilon/\delta\right)^2 + 4/\delta\right]^{0.5} \qquad (3)$$

where $\delta = 2.77 \, (f/\Delta f)^2$, $\epsilon = 0.115 R f_t \alpha$, R is the range of the sample volume, and α the attenuation coefficient in dB MHz^{-1} cm^{-1}. The ratio of f_d'/f_d is plotted as a function of $R f_t \alpha$ in *figure 15.2*. It can be seen that the effects of frequency dependent mechanisms become significant only for very short pulses.

15.3.3 Spectral analysis limitations

Spectral analysis of Doppler signals has already been discussed in the section on CW Doppler. There are however two extra limitations to be considered with PW Doppler. The first is that there is no point in sampling the signal at a rate greater

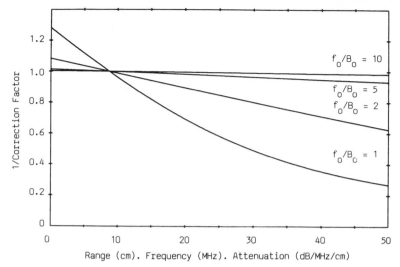

Figure 15.2 The Doppler correction factor (i.e. the error introduced into the mean Doppler shift by frequency dependent mechanisms) as derived by Newhouse (*reference 13*).

than the transmission pulse repetition frequency, the second is that there is no advantage to be gained from using an analysing resolution Δf_a of less than Δf_{tt}, the spectral width of the Doppler signal that results from a single scatterer. Short pulses lead to large values of Δf_{tt}, and if $1/\Delta f_{tt}$ is larger than T_s the period of stationarity it is better to reduce the spectral variance by performing a number of spectral estimations on short data segments.

15.3.4 Velocity limit

Because the Doppler waveform is reconstructed from a series of samples taken at regular intervals in PW techniques, there is a maximum Doppler shift f_{max} which can be unambiguously detected. This is normally equal to half the pulse repetition frequency ($f_p/2$), but it is sometimes possible to increase this to f_p if it is known that the flow is undirectional. Assuming the former criterion obtains, the maximum velocity that can be detected by a PW unit can be found by rewriting equation 1 in terms of f_p:

$$v_{max} = (f_p\, c)/(4\, f_t \cos \theta) \qquad (4)$$

When the velocity exceeds this limit then aliasing occurs, and f_p is subtracted from f_d. If the velocity continues to increase then the apparent velocity rises from $-v_{max}$ to $+v_{max}$ until once again the frequency flips over. Aliasing is a fundamental limitation of pulsed systems and can only be overcome by increasing f_p.

15.3.5 Velocity-range limit

The position of the range gate in a PW system is determined by the time delay between transmission and commencement of signal acquisition. In principle there is always range ambiguity since the signals arriving at a given time can be the

124

results of echoes from the current pulse, the previous pulse or even earlier pulses. Signals are therefore collected from ranges given by:

$$z = (c/2) (T_d + n T_p) \tag{5}$$

where n is any non-negative integer. In practice, because of attenuation, the signals returning from deeper tissues are much weaker, and if f_p is low, negligible. There are thus two conflicting requirements for f_p; if velocity ambiguity is to be avoided it must be high, and if range ambiguity is to be avoided it should be as low as possible. The maximum range z_{max} from which pulses return during the same transmission cycle is given by:

$$z_{max} = c \, T_p/2 \tag{6}$$

Combining this equation with equation 4 leads to the relationship:

$$v_{max} \cdot z_{max} = c^2/8 \, f_t \cos \theta \tag{7}$$

This equation shows that the product of the maximum observable velocity and maximum range is limited in conventional PW systems, but equation 7 can only be used as a rough guide since neither type of ambiguity can be totally eliminated. In practice range ambiguity is not usually a serious problem, except possibly in the heart, because, providing the sites of the range gates are known, care can be taken to ensure that only one of them encompasses a vessel.

15.4 Conclusion

Doppler ultrasound is a relatively simple technique to use, but care must be taken with the interpretation of results obtained using CW and particulary PW techniques. The instantaneous power spectrum reflects, to a first approximation, the velocity distribution of the erythrocytes within the sample volume of the device, but it is only an approximation for the several reasons discussed above. *Table 15.1* summarises some of the relative merits of the CW and the PW techniques.

Table 15.1 Comparison between continuous wave and pulsed wave doppler.

CONTINUOUS WAVE	PULSED WAVE
Simple	Range resolution (but possible ambiguity)
No range resolution	Limit on maximum velocity
No limit on maximum measurable velocity	Possibly significant spectral broadening

References

1 SATOMURA S 1957 Ultrasonic Doppler method for the inspection of cardiac function *J Acoust Soc Am* **29** 1181–1185
2 EVANS D H 1982 Some aspects of the relationship between instantaneous volumetric blood flow and continuous wave Doppler ultrasound recordings — III. The calculation of Doppler power spectra from mean velocity waveforms, and the results of processing these with maximum, mean, and RMS frequency processors *Ultrasound Med Biol* **8** 617–623

3   EVANS D H 1985 On the measurement of the mean velocity of blood flow over the cardiac cycle using Doppler ultrasound *Ultrasound Med Biol* **11** 735–741

4   EVANS D H and PARTON L 1981 The directional characteristics of some ultrasonic Doppler blood flow probes *Ultrasound Med Biol* **7** 51–62

5   DOUVILLE Y, ARENSON J W, JOHNSON K W, COBBOLD R S C and KASSAM M 1983 Critical evaluation of continuous wave Doppler probes for carotid studies *J Clin Ultrasound* **11** 83–90

6   SHUNG K K, SIGELMANN R A and REID J M 1976 Scattering of ultrasound by blood *IEEE Trans Biomed Engng* **BME–23** 460–467

7   ANGELSEN B A J 1980 A theoretical study of the scattering of ultrasound from blood *IEEE Trans Biomed Engng* **BME–27** 61–67

8   COBBOLD R S C, VELTINK P H and JOHNSTON K W 1983 Influence of beam profile and degree of insonation on the CW Doppler ultrasound spectrum and mean velocity *IEEE Trans Sonics Ultrason* **SU–30** 364–370

9   GERZBERG L and MEINDL J D 1977 Mean frequency estimator with applications in ultrasonic Doppler flowmeters *Ultrasound in medicine* **3B** 1173–1180, (Eds D White and R E Brown) (Plenum Press, New York)

10 GILL R W 1979 Performance of the mean frequency Doppler modulator *Ultrasound Med Biol* **5** 237–247

11 KINSLER L E and FREY A R 1962 *Fundamentals of acoustics* p 166 (Wiley, New York)

12 STEPANISHEN P R 1971 Transient radiation from pistons in an infinite planar baffle *J Acoust Soc Am* **49** 1629–1638

13 NEWHOUSE V L, EHRENWALD A R and JOHNSON G F 1977 The effect of Rayleigh scattering and frequency dependent absorption on the output spectrum of Doppler flowmeters *Ultrasound in Medicine* **3B** 1181–1191 (Eds D White and R E Brown) (Plenum Press, New York)

CHAPTER 16

Towards Real-Time Classification of Doppler Waveforms

S B Sherriff and D C Barber
Department of Medical Physics and Clinical Engineering, Royal Hallamshire Hospital, Sheffield S10 2JF

16.1 Introduction

In the past it has been shown that mathematical feature extraction techniques applied to the Doppler shifted signal from the common carotid artery offer an accurate objective method of signal analysis and patient classification[1,2]. In this previous work a principal components analysis followed by a data classification was performed off-line on both the maximum frequency envelope (MFE) and the total waveform. Such off-line methods are of little use in routine diagnosis and recently we have developed a micro-computer based system for objective analysis of signal waveforms on-line. The aim of this paper is to show that by careful design of the complete algorithm, apparently sophisticated techniques of analysis can nevertheless be used for rapid 'near real-time' data classification.

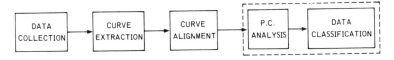

Figure 16.1 Principal features of a real-time system for analysis of Doppler waveforms.

16.2 Data collection

The basis of a real-time system is shown in *figure 16.1*. Following collection of the Doppler signal, directional demodulation and frequency analysis, the data is typically in the form of 128 frequency points representing a digitisation rate of 12.8 ms per spectrum. In order to keep the number of bits used to a minimum, while preserving low amplitude signals, the frequency analyser currently being used computes the square root of the frequency amplitude information before quantisation to 4 bits; this data must be squared to produce an estimate of the orginal frequency amplitude, giving 'pseudo 8 bit' non-linearly quantised data. Preliminary results suggest that the effect of this non-linear quantisation on classification efficiency is negligible. On completion of each FFT the signal from the frequency analyser is transferred into a Z80 micro-computer.

16.3 Waveform analysis

16.3.1 Waveform extraction

In this work the median frequency, the 25th and the 75th percentile frequencies are extracted from each FFT. From the median and these percentiles a maximum frequency envelope value is computed by the following formulae:

$$MFE = Median + 2.25\,(M75 - Median) \quad Median > 0 \quad\quad (1a)$$
$$MFE = Median + 2.25\,(M25 - Median) \quad Median < 0 \quad\quad (1b)$$
$$MFE = Median \quad\quad\quad\quad\quad\quad\quad\quad\quad\quad Median = 0 \quad\quad (1c)$$

where M25 is the 25th frequency percentile and M75 is the 75th frequency percentile. The median and these percentiles are used in preference to other measures in this real-time system because they can be rapidly computed without extensive use of multiplication and division. Ten sets of values representing 128 ms of data are stored at any one time in a rolling buffer until the onset of a cycle is detected in the median waveform. The onset of a waveform is detected by the value of the median waveform exceeding an operator chosen threshold. This threshold can be adjusted by the operator at any time during the investigation. A further 54 spectra are collected and analysed after the threshold is detected and are then concatenated with the 10 existing sets of values to complete a waveform of 64 points representing a total of 820 ms of data.

16.3.2 Waveform alignment

In the analysis of these waveforms by principal components factor analysis it is essential to remove non-significant waveform variations from the data before analysis. It is assumed that the overall width of the pulsatile part of the waveform

Curve Standardisation

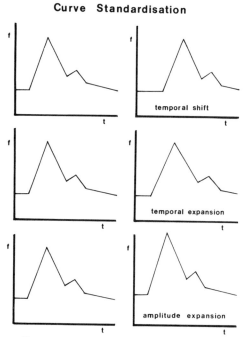

Figure 16.2 Curve alignment and standardisation (a) temporal shift, (b) temporal expansion, and (c) amplitude expansion.

and the delay between each heart contraction and the initial rise of the pulse are controlled by factors not relevant to the shape of the waveform. In addition the position of the pulsatile part of the waveform within the 64 data points collected will also depend slightly on the value of the detection threshold. It is assumed that the strength of the signal is dependent on, or cannot be separated from, physical factors such as the angle of insonation.

The alignment technique used in this work is simpler than that previously published and is shown diagrammatically in *figure 16.2*. The time average T and the half width W of the pulsatile part of the median waveform are computed after subtraction of the diastolic flow level and these measures are used to transform the maximum frequency waveform to standard form using the two parameter warp given by

$$t' = \frac{(t - T_s)\, W}{W_s} + T \tag{2}$$

where T_s and W_s are standard values, t is the time coordinate of the shifted waveform being generated and t' is the time coordinate of the value of the waveform to be moved to t. t' is generally not an integer value and the waveform value at t' is extracted by linear interpolation between the two nearest neighbours. The significance of this transformation is that if it were applied to the median waveform the values of T and W for this waveform would then assume the standard values T_s and W_s. Once position and width have been fixed each signal is scaled in amplitude to bring its average value to a standard value.

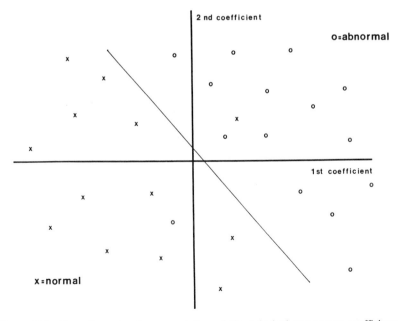

Figure 16.3 Two dimensional representation of the principal component coefficients together with a separating plane.

16.3.3 Principal components and classification

The best single waveform classification is obtained using the maximum frequency envelope. In the current system five coefficients for the MFE can be extracted using the principal components previously computed from a mixed sample of normal and abnormal waveforms. The five coefficients computed for each patient represent a point in five dimensional space. Coefficients from normal signals tend to plot in one region of this space and coefficients from abnormal signals tend to plot in a second region. A simple two dimensional analogue of this is shown in *figure 16.3*. A plane can be found which optimally separates these regions and the normal distance d of a point to the plane can be determined using the formula

$$d = \vec{c}.\bar{w} - w_0 \qquad (3)$$

where $\vec{c}$ is a (row) vector of the coefficients of the waveform (a five dimensional vector in the present case) and $\bar{w}$ is the (column) vector representing the unit normal to the separating plane. w_0 is the distance from the origin of the space to the separating plane. The sign of d is an indication of which side of the line the point lies and hence into which group the curve is to be classified. In this paper a positive value of d signifies classification into the normal group.

The value of w_0, μ and the elements of $\bar{w}$ may be determined using a function minimisation procedure which minimises F in equation 4d given

$$C(d) = 1 - \exp(-\mu.d) \qquad\qquad d > 0 \qquad (4a)$$
$$C(d) = \quad 0 \qquad\qquad\qquad\qquad d = 0 \qquad (4b)$$
$$C(d) = \exp(\mu.d) - 1 \qquad\qquad d < 0 \qquad (4c)$$

$$F = \sum_{\substack{\text{normal}\\\text{group}}} (1 - C(d))^2 \quad + \sum_{\substack{\text{abnormal}\\\text{group}}} (1 + C(d))^2 \qquad (4d)$$

where d is given by equation 3.

The value of G in

$$G = 0.5 \exp(-\mu.d) \qquad\qquad d > 0 \qquad (5a)$$
$$G = 0.5 \qquad\qquad\qquad\qquad d = 0 \qquad (5b)$$
$$G = 1.0 - 0.5 \exp(\mu.d) \qquad\qquad d < 0 \qquad (5c)$$

can then be taken as a measure of membership of the abnormal group in a fuzzy set sense[3] or as an indication of the certainty of the point classification.

Finally it can be shown that the extraction of the coefficients and the calculation of d can be merged into one single step. In this work normalised coefficients are used for classification so the value of the ith element of $\vec{c}$ is given by

$$c_i = \frac{(\vec{g} - \vec{m}).\vec{e}_i}{L_i^{1/2}} \qquad (6)$$

where $\vec{g}$ is the waveform, $\vec{m}$ is the mean waveform of the population of waveforms used to compute the principal components, $\vec{e}_i$ is the ith principal

130

component and L_i is the ith eigenvalue. Then substituting equation 6 into equation 3 gives after some reduction

$$d = \vec{g} \cdot \vec{s} - \vec{m} \cdot \vec{s} - w_0 \tag{7}$$

where $\vec{s}$ is a classification factor given by

$$\vec{s} = \sum_{\text{all } i} \frac{w_i \cdot \vec{e}_i}{L_i^{1/2}} \tag{8}$$

The last two terms in equation 7 may be precomputed so that classification of the waveform $\vec{g}$ reduces to evaluation of the scalar product $\vec{g} \cdot \vec{s}$.

The classification factor $\vec{s}$ represents the normal to the separating plane transformed back into the space of the original waveforms $\vec{g}$. Interpretation of the significance of the principal components is often difficult since principal components describe overall shape variations irrespective of whether these are of diagnostic significance or not. The classification factor however can be used to identify those differences in curve shape which distinguish between normal and abnormal waveforms. Inspection of the classification factor of *figure 16.4* suggests that the slope of the initial upswing of the waveform and the difference between the amplitude of the A and B peaks of the waveform are both significant in classifying these waveforms.

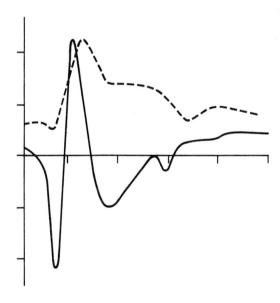

Figure 16.4 The classification factor (—) computed as in the text from a population of normal and abnormal carotid waveforms, a typical normal waveform is also shown (---).

16.4 Implementation

The processes outlined above can be divided into three stages. These are:

(a) Data collection and waveform extraction.
(b) Waveform alignment.
(c) Waveform classification.

Transfer of each FFT, and extraction of the median and the 25th and 75th percentiles takes less than 12.8 ms on the micro-processor used and so waveform extraction can be performed during data collection. These operations are written in assembly code. Collection of a full 64 point waveform takes 820 ms. Waveform alignment and classification together take approximately a further 500 ms giving a total analysis time from the beginning of data acquisition of between 1.3 and 1.4 seconds which usually allows analysis of every other waveform. The data collection system is at present not interrupt driven and hardware multiply and divide is not available. Addition of these two features could significantly reduce the total time for analysis. Construction of a simple two processor system, one for collection and one for analysis could produce a system capable of analysing every waveform.

16.5 Other features

Each waveform successfully detected is displayed on the system VDU as shown in *figure 16.5*. The displayed curve is the current MFE being analysed. As well as two

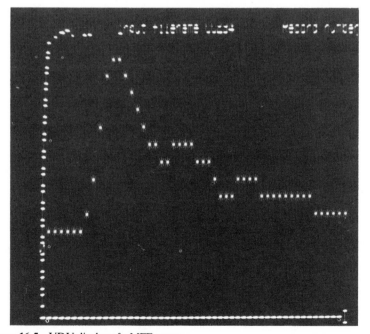

Figure 16.5   VDU display of a MFE curve.

132

other flow indices the abnormality index given by 100.G is also shown on the screen. Once the optimum display and threshold levels have been established no further action is required by the operator. Acquisition of data may be suspended at any time simply by lifting the Doppler probe from the investigation site and restablished by restoring the probe and obtaining a good signal.

The system stores within memory the last four waveforms and these may be reviewed and archived to disk as required. A separate recall and review program is available for post-investigation study of the waveforms.

16.6 Conclusion

Although classification of carotid waveforms by principal components analysis appears to be a fairly sophisticated approach we have shown that by careful design of the appropriate algorithms it is possible to produce a near real-time on-line system for analysis of these waveforms.

References

1   MARTIN T R P, BARBER D C, SHERRIFF S B and PRICHARD D R 1980 Objective feature extraction applied to the diagnosis of carotid disease using a Doppler ultrasound technique *Clin Phys Physiol Meas* **1** 71–81
2   SHERRIFF S B, BARBER D C, MARTIN T R P and LAKEMAN J M 1982 The use of principal component factor analysis in the detection of carotid artery disease from Doppler ultrasound *Med Biol Eng Comp* **20** 351–356
3   ZADEH L A 1965 Fuzzy Sets *Inf Control* **8** 338–353

CHAPTER 17

Quantitative Doppler with Ultrasound Pulses

S Leeman, V C Roberts and K Willson*
Department of Medical Engineering and Physics, King's College School of Medicine and Dentistry, Denmark Hill, London SE5, and
**Bioengineering Department, St Thomas's Hospital, Lambeth Palace Road, London SE1 7EH*

17.1 Introduction

The use of pulsed fields in Doppler studies is necessitated by the growing need for simultaneous range and velocity discrimination in many medical ultrasound applications. Much of the conceptual basis for, and, indeed, the formulation of, the Doppler effect and its applications has been in terms of monochromatic, continuous, plane-wave fields. Some of these concepts are no longer valid when applied blindly to investigations with (wide-band) pulses. Moreover, the physics of pulse propagation and scattering in human tissues is not necessarily easily derivable from a consideration of individual spectral components. Many of the difficulties are better understood by considering a time-domain formulation of the Doppler principle, and by bearing in mind the intricacies of pulse transmission and scattering. Only in this way will the pulse Doppler technique evolve into a truly quantitative velocity estimation method.

17.2 The Doppler effect for transient fields

The well-known Doppler effect may be somewhat generally characterised as being the apparent change of wave frequency (as perceived by some observer) which results from relative motion between the wave source and that observer. When applied to pulsed fields, concepts such a 'frequency of the wave' become rather fuzzy, and recourse must be made to the Fourier domain for rigorous clarification. Since the Doppler effect is a real phenomenon, its expression should not be dependent on such abstract notions as Fourier space, and we investigate whether there is a simple and direct formulation of the Doppler effect in terms of time-domain concepts alone. Such an approach is bound to be of value in analysing the problems of quantitative velocity measurement with ultrasound pulses, via the Doppler effect.

Consider the one-dimensional pulse, $f(t)$, which may be expressed in terms of its Fourier transform, $F(w)$, as follows:

$$f(t) = (1/2\pi) \int_{-\infty}^{\infty} dw\, F(w)\, \exp(iwt) \qquad (1)$$

Here, t denotes time and w (circular) frequency. The 'Doppler shifted' version of the pulse, $f_D(t)$, is the pulse which results when each of its Fourier components undergoes an appropriate frequency shift. For the case that $f_D(t)$ represents the pulse (as perceived) from a source moving with velocity v (assumed positive for an approaching, and negative for a receding, source), each frequency, w, shifts to a new value, $w' = w/(1-\beta)$, with $\beta=v/c$, where c is the ultrasound velocity in the (static) intervening medium. The Doppler-shifted waveform can be written as

$$f_D(t) = (1/2\pi) \int_{-\infty}^{\infty} dw'\, F_D(w') \exp(iw't)$$
$$= (1/2\pi) \int_{-\infty}^{\infty} dw\, F(w) \exp[iwt/(1-\beta)] \qquad (2)$$

since the Doppler effect implies the transformation

$$F(w)dw \;\rightarrow\; F_D(w')dw'$$

Equation (2) is the statement that

$$f_D(t) = f(t/[1-\beta])$$

Thus, in the time domain, the Doppler effect may be characterised as the apparent change in wave time-scale (as perceived by some observer) which results from relative motion between the wave source and that observer. This formulation is particularly suited to the consideration of transient fields.

The signals generated in medical ultrasound applications may, quite generally, be represented as

$$f(t) = a(t)\, \cos[\phi(t)]$$

where $a(t)$ denotes the envelope (always presumed ≥ 0), and $\phi(t)$ the signal phase. This type of one-dimensional representation applies to a very wide class of 'practical' signals, and there are prescriptions for unambiguously determining both envelope and phase, individually, once the signal, $f(t)$, is specified. The time-derivative of the phase function is defined as the instantaneous, or temporal, (circular) frequency, which is denoted here by $\dot\phi(t)$. Clearly, the instantaneous frequency is time-dependent in general, and, as even a very simple example will show, is certainly not equal to the Fourier domain frequency of the signal, except for the special case that $\phi=\phi_o + w_ot$, with $a=$constant. The essential difference between instantaneous and 'Fourier' frequency has not been appreciated in most fundamental treatments of Doppler ultrasound methods[1,2].

17.3   Time- and Fourier-domain methods

Consider the simple one-dimensional case of an emitted pulse of the form

$$f_e(t) = A_o \cos(\nu_o t) \qquad 0 \leq t \leq 2T_o$$
$$= 0 \qquad \text{otherwise}$$

Time-domain arguments predict that the pulse reflected from a rigid interface travelling with constant velocity, v, towards the emitter, is of the form

$$f_r(t) = -A_o \cos[\nu(t-\tau)] \qquad 0 \leq (t-\tau) \leq 2T$$
$$= 0 \qquad \text{otherwise}$$

135

where τ denotes the delay in receiving the reflected pulse, and the Doppler principle demands that

$$(\nu - \nu_o)/\nu_o = 2v/c$$

and $\qquad T = T_o(1-2v/c)$

Ideal transfer characteristics of the receiver are assumed throughout. A fairly straightforward Fourier analysis reveals that, provided $\nu_o >> 2\pi/T_o$, then the power spectrum of the emitted pulse, for $w > 0$, is

$$P_e(w) = A_o^2 \sin^2[T_o(w-\nu_o)] / (w-\nu_o)^2$$

with $\qquad \bar{w}_e = \nu_o$

For the received pulse

$$P_r(w) = A_o^2 \sin^2[T_o(1-2\beta)(w-\nu_o/(1-2\beta))] \cdot [w-\nu_o/(1-2\beta)]^{-2}$$

with $\qquad \bar{w}_r = \nu_o/(1-2\beta)$

The mean spectral frequencies are defined as

$$\bar{w}_s = \int_o^\alpha wP_s(w)\, dw / \int_o^\alpha P_s(w)\, dw \qquad s=e, r$$

It is clear, from the spectral distributions, that negative frequency 'shifts' ($w < \nu_o$) do not necessarily imply negative Doppler shifts! The interface velocity may, however, be recovered from the mean frequencies,

$$v/c = (\bar{w}_r - \bar{w}_e)/2\bar{w}_e$$

An important conclusion to be made from consideration of this simple example is the very clear demonstration that, given the power spectra of single emitted and received pulses (as obtained by processing of digitised signals, for example), there is, in principle, no range-velocity limitation. That is, the velocity of the interface is in principle obtainable with a single emitted pulse (PRF=0 !), and there is no upper limit to the velocity that can thereby be measured, at any range. The range-velocity relation that may be (mis)construed as a fundamental limitation of pulse Doppler methods[1,2] is, in fact, a consequence of the particular (hardware) processing method that is used to measure the Doppler shift.

These somewhat unexpected findings may be emphasised by considering the above example from the point of view of instantaneous frequency measurement. For the signals considered in this case, the instantaneous frequency may be shown to be that measured by a zero-crossing detector, but, in general, the ϕ values should be preferably recovered via digital processing.

For the emitted pulse,

$$\phi_e(t) = \nu_o \qquad \text{(constant)}$$

and for the received echo,

$$\phi_r(t) = \nu \qquad \text{(constant)}$$

Hence

$$v/c = (\phi_r - \phi_e)/2\phi_e$$

The result is again, in principle, obtainable with a single pulse-echo sequence (i.e. PRF=0), and there is no fundamental range-velocity limitation. Note also that the time-domain technique is actually independent of pulse shape (envelope). It should be clear also that the time domain provides the simpler approach towards analysing the example presented here. The pulses considered in this section possess the fortuitous property that $\phi = \bar{w}$: this does not hold in general.

17.4 Problems with quantitative pulse Doppler

In practice, a number of factors intrude, which militate against achieving the quantitative velocity estimates obtained in the idealised example of the previous section. These artefacts are generated by effects associated both with the propagation of pulses in real media, and also with the scattering (reflection) of pulses from real tissue inhomogeneities.

17.4.1 Propagation effects: attenuation downshifts

Treatments of Doppler methods neglect to take into account the frequency-dependent nature of the attenuation coefficient, $\alpha(w)$, of human tissues. In practice, it has been observed that a useful parametrisation of $\alpha(w)$, in the diagnostic frequency range, is

$$\alpha(w) = \alpha_0 w^n \qquad \text{with } n \approx 1, \quad \alpha_0 \text{ constant}$$

Other parametrisations are equally valid, but many pulse-echo attenuation estimation techniques assume the above, with $n=1$ (*reference 3*). The exact nature of the frequency dependence is uncertain, but experiments leave little doubt that attenuation rises with frequency: thus, a propagating pulse has its higher frequency components preferentially attenuated, with the result that its mean frequency is progressively downshifted with depth. Thus, since the Doppler shift depends on the pulse spectrum actually incident on the moving scatterer, and since the Doppler-shifted echo is likewise downshifted on its return path to the transducer, quantitative velocity assessments will be difficult unless the frequency dependence of the attenuation of the intervening medium is known. Note that the magnitude of the artefact increases with the range of the scatterer, and with the bandwidth of the emitted pulse. The magnitude of the artefact is relatively easily demonstrated by considering a pulse of the form $\exp[-b^2t^2].\cos(\nu_0 t)$ propagating from location $x=0$ to $x=L$, through a uniform medium with attenuation $\alpha(w) = \alpha_0 w$. Such a gaussian pulse is not physically exactly realisable, but may be closely approximated in practice. The initial mean frequency of the pulse is ν_0, but after propagation through the distance L, the mean frequency is downshifted to $\nu_0 - 2b^2\alpha_0 L$. Insertion of some typical values will demonstrate that attenuation downshifts may cause significant artefacts in quantitative pulse Doppler studies.

17.4.2 Propagation effects: diffraction

Real pulses are not one-dimensional entities, but consist of bounded, three-dimensional packets of acoustical energy. The structure of these pulses is heavily modified by phenomena associated with the finite size of the transducer apertures utilised in all applications. These 'diffraction effects' may be shown to arise from the edges (boundaries) of the transmitting transducer for propagation in lossless media, with more subtle features operating in lossy media[4]. As a consequence, the pressure waveform experienced by a small scatterer, located within the path of the pulse, may vary quite significantly throughout the field. Since the same holds for both the mean and instantaneous frequencies perceived by the scatterer, an apparently location-dependent Doppler shift will be registered. Diffraction effects come into play also when a transducer acts in reception mode, thus exaggerating the artefact. Diffraction has come under considerable study for its adverse influence when measuring attenuation by backscattering, and a random selection from the published literature[5] will indicate the large magnitude this artefact can assume in certain cases.

17.4.3 Non-linear propagation effects

The propagation of ultrasound waves in all real media is governed by non-linear laws, but it is common practice to invoke the acoustic wave equation in its linear approximation only. One consequence of non-linearity is that entities such as wave velocity and attenuation would be found to have values that depend on the amplitude of the ultrasound wave. Another, perhaps more important, effect is that the lower frequency components of the pulse act as 'sources' which (non-linearly) pump energy into higher frequencies, thereby leading, initially, to a progressive increase of pulse mean frequency with depth. However, as the pulse becomes more attenuated, and its intensity drops, the effect diminishes, as the linear propagation approximation becomes valid. Non-linear propagation can generate a number of quite subtle effects, and it is difficult to make a general estimate of these hitherto neglected artefacts in Doppler investigations.

17.4.4 Scattering effects: interference

Interference of pulses scattered or reflected from closely-spaced inhomogeneities can give rise to very large excursions of the instantaneous frequency, irrespective of whether the echoes are Doppler shifted, or not. These ϕ-fluctuations can be of either sign, and interference is one of the most significant artefacts confusing quantitative Doppler measurements by an instantaneous frequency approach. Mean frequencies may similarly be affected: consider the simple case of a one-dimensional pulse reflected from two stationary, identical reflectors, separated by a distance L. If the Fourier spectrum of the echo from the proximal reflector is F(w), then the Fourier spectrum of the echo sequence from the two reflectors is given by

$$F_2(w) = F(w) + \exp[iwL] \, F(w)$$

The power spectrum of the echo pair is easily shown to be

$$| F_2(w) |^2 = 4 | F(w) |^2 \cos^2 (wL/2) \tag{3}$$

It is clear that the mean frequency of the echo pair may deviate (positively or negatively) from the mean frequency of a single echo. Such deviations would be misinterpreted, in practice, as (artefactual) Doppler shifts. Note how Equation (3) emphasises the hazards of associating mean frequency shift with mean velocity (ie. velocity weighted by the relative distribution of material moving at that speed). Certainly, in this case, despite the assumption of no multiple scattering, the total scattered power spectrum from the group of scatterers need not be the sum of the powers returned by each scatterer (in isolation).

17.4.5 Frequency-dependent scattering

Reflection and, in particular, scattering processes may be strongly frequency dependent. Indeed, the intensity of scattering from blood shows a w^4-dependence (Rayleigh scattering) at lower haematocrit values[2]. Assume that the scattering law is of the general form S(w), where experiments would suggest that S(w) is monotonically increasing with w, in the diagnostic frequency range. An incident pulse with Fourier spectrum F(w) would be scattered to form an observed echo with Fourier spectrum S(w).F(w), and with mean frequency clearly shifted upwards with respect to that for the incident pulse, even in the absence of any relative motion. Our calculations suggest that this artefact is significant for Rayleigh scattering of broadband pulses. Although such scattering phenomena are usually described in the Fourier domain, the instantaneous frequency of the echo is also affected.

17.5 Conclusions

The formulation of the Doppler effect in the time domain emphasises the advantages of the instantaneous frequency concept in certain cases. Analysis of a simple example demonstrated that the range-velocity limitation is not fundamental to pulse Doppler studies, and that it may be overcome by, for example, digital processing methods. On the other hand, a variety of artefacts are injected by the physics of pulse propagation and scattering. Significant, but artefactual, frequency shifts may be generated by effects associated with frequency-dependent attenuation, diffraction, pulse interference, and frequency-dependent scattering. Non-linear propagation effects are more difficult to estimate, but may well be significant in certain cases. In practice, interference artefacts may be reduced by the gross statistical averaging occurring when pulses interact with the large numbers of cells in blood. Moreover, the mean frequency downshifts caused by attenuation may well be partially counterbalanced by the frequency upshifts resulting from the Rayleigh-like scattering by blood cells. Diffraction effects may be virtually eliminated by the use of appropriate transducers[6]. Certainly, qualitative pulse Doppler methods work well in the clinic, and provide much useful information. However, the artefacts we have reported on here (some of which do not appear to have been raised in a Doppler context before) need to be constantly borne in mind when interpreting data from which truly quantitative information is desired.

References

1   ATKINSON P and WOODCOCK J P 1982 *Doppler Ultrasound and its use in Clinical Measurement* (Academic Press: London)
2   BAKER D W, FORSTER F K and DAIGLE R E 1978 Doppler principles and techniques In: *Ultrasound: Its Applications in Medicine and Biology*, (Ed. F J Fry) 161 (Elsevier: Amsterdam)
3   LEEMAN S, FERRARI L A, JONES J P and FINK M 1984 Perspectives on attenuation estimation from pulse-echo signals *IEEE Trans Sonics and Ultrasonics* **SU–31** 352
4   LEEMAN S, HUTCHINS L and JONES J P 1982 Bounded pulse propagation In: *Acoustical Imaging 10*, (Eds. P Alais and A F Metherell), 427 (Plenum: New York)

5   O'DONNELL M 1983 Effects of diffraction on measurements of the frequency dependent ultrasonic attenuation *IEEE Trans Biomed Eng* **BME–30**/6 320

6   LEEMAN S, SEGGIE D, FERRARI L A, SANKAR P V and DOHERTY M 1985 Diffraction-free attenuation estimation *Proc Ultrasonics Int '85*, (Ed. Z Novak) In Press (Butterworth: Sevenoaks)

CHAPTER 18

A New Technique to Measure Blood Flow using Doppler Ultrasound

J M Evans, R Skidmore and P N T Wells
Department of Medical Physics, Level 7, Bristol Royal Infirmary, Bristol BS2 8HW

18.1 Introduction

Doppler ultrasound has been used non-invasively to measure volume blood flow by estimating the product of mean blood velocity and lumen area[1]. The measurement of the lumen area is obtained by observing the vessel diameter or cross-section by means of a pulse-echo ultrasound imaging system. The computation of the mean velocity requires even insonation of the blood-vessel, the estimate of beam vessel angle and the evaluation of the first moment of the Doppler power spectrum.

The majority of volume flow estimates have been achieved using duplex systems. Since these scanners are optimised for imaging, they do not provide a beam which is sufficiently wide for complete, even insonation. Moreover, the estimations of the beam-vessel angle and lumen area, especially with deep lying vessels, are the largest sources of error with this technique[2].

An alternative method of estimating blood volume flow rate non-invasively has been proposed[3] which does not require estimation of the angle of insonation or lumen area.

18.2 Attenuation compensated approach

This relatively new and unexplored method called the Attenuation Compensated Volume Flowmeter (ACVF) consists of a two parallel channel pulsed Doppler system using two concentric ultrasound beams. The first is a wide beam whose sample volume totally encompasses the vessel lumen. The backscattered Doppler power is then proportional to the projected lumen area and the first moment of the Doppler power spectrum represents the projected instantaneous mean velocity through the projected area. The resultant product is then proportional to volume flow rate which in this case is independent of beam vessel angle and lumen area (*figure 18.1*).

However, absolute volume flow rate cannot be determined from this product alone since factors such as ultrasonic attenuation in tissue and the scattering efficiency of blood are not known. By using the second of the two concentric ultrasound beams, these unknown factors (K) can be indirectly found. An absolute measure of volume flow rate is then the product of the mean frequency of the wide beam and the ratio of the returned powers from both ultrasonic beams once the range dependent calibration constant (Kc) has been determined (*figure 18.2*). This approach assumes that the backscattered power from moving blood is independent of blood velocity and does not fluctuate. Initial results from *in-vitro* flow tank experiments show that the power is independent of velocity provided

141

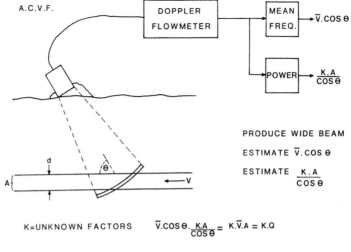

Figure 18.1 The product of mean frequency and backscattered power is proportional to flow.

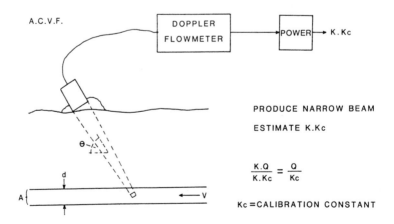

Figure 18.2 An absolute measurement of flow can be made after the range dependent calibration constant has been determined.

that sufficient time-averaging of the Doppler power signal is employed to smooth the fluctuation of the Doppler signal.

18.3   System design

The main practical problem in implementing this technique is that of producing a wide enough beam in order to achieve lateral even insonation. For example, the measurement of cardiac output from the suprasternal notch requires a beam width of 30 mm at a distance of 50 mm from the transducer face. Initial work using a four element annular array at 3 MHz has shown that it is possible to produce both a wide and a narrow beam from the same transducer by choosing the appropriate aperture function in terms of amplitude and phase. However, acceptable results have been obtained from a 2 MHz two element annular array. At a depth of 50 mm the 3 dB beam width ratio of the two beams is approximately three to one, the wide beam being 24 mm.

A two channel directional pulsed Doppler system has been constructed with the gain and phase of each transmitter and receiver adjustable (*figure 18.3*). Switched capacitor filters were incorporated to obtain variable wall filter, pulse repetition frequency and gate length. The transmit and receive aperture functions may be adjusted for different depths of interest and the overall pulsed Doppler system has been designed to be totally controlled by a microcomputer.

An analogue mean frequency estimator[4] is employed to calculate the first moment of the Doppler power spectrum and analogue multipliers followed by low pass filters used to determine the backscattered Doppler power from the two beams. The final computation of time-averaged volume flow is achieved by the microcomputer.

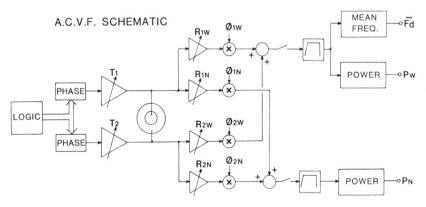

Figure 18.3   By adjusting the gain (T and R) and phase (ϕ) the appropriate aperture function is produced.

18.4   In-vitro results

Citrated whole human blood at room temperature, haematocrit 40 per cent, was pumped through a 15 mm thin-walled plastic tube in series with an in-line electromagnetic flow probe at flow rates up to 1500 ml min^{-1}. The electromagnetic flowmeter had been previously calibrated by timed flow of blood into a measuring cylinder and was found to be linear within one per cent over the flow range of interest. The plastic tube was submerged in a tank of water and the two element array probe suspended 50 mm above at a known angle.

The power ratio was found to be constant to within four per cent over the flow range 1000 ml min^{-1} to 1500 ml min^{-1} at an angle of 55 degrees. With a constant flow rate of 1500 ml min^{-1} the angle of insonation was then varied between 45 degrees and 70 degrees with the resultant ACVF flow being constant to within eight per cent.

The former result validates one of the assumptions that backscattered power remains constant with velocity and the latter result indicates that the power ratio is proportional to the insonated flow area.

To test the system for attenuation compensation, an attenuation medium was placed between the transducer array and the tube. The resultant ACVF flow varied by only two per cent with a change in returned power of 6 dB.

The ACVF flow was found to be linear within five per cent of the measured electromagnetic flow over the flow range 800 ml min^{-1} to 1500 ml min^{-1}.

18.5 Conclusion

By using an annular array transducer, wide and narrow pulsed Doppler beam shapes can be formed. The beam shape ratio is approximately three to one with a two element array but can be improved by using a larger number of elements at the expense of increased complexity of Doppler electronics.

The backscattered power ratio from blood has been shown to be constant with flow and also proportional to lumen area.

The ACVF has been shown to be independent of beam-vessel angle and attenuation and has the potential to measure volume flow non-invasively independent of lumen area and angle of insonation.

References

1   GILL R W 1979 Pulsed Doppler with B-mode imaging for quantitative blood flow measurements *Ultrasound in Medicine and Biology* **5** 223–235
2   GILL R W 1982 Accuracy calculations for ultrasonic pulsed Doppler blood flow measurements *Australasian Physical and Engineering Sciences in Medicine* **5** 51–57
3   HOTTINGER C F and MEINDL J D 1979 Blood flow measurement using the attenuation compensated volume flowmeter *Ultrasonic Imaging* **1** 1–15
4   EVANS J M, SKIDMORE R, WOODCOCK J P and BURNS P N 1982 Measurement of blood flow using ultrasound In *Acoustical Imaging* **12** (Eds E A Ash and C R Hill) pp 539–546 (Plenum Press, New York)

CHAPTER 19

Can Ultrasonic Duplex Scanners Really Measure Volumetric Flow?

D H Evans
Department of Medical Physics and Clinical Engineering, Leicester Royal Infirmary, Leicester LE1 5WW

19.1 Introduction

A number of ultrasonic duplex scanners (scanners which combine a real-time pulse-echo imaging system with a pulsed or continuous wave Doppler system) now have facilities for calculating and displaying mean flow rates in intact blood vessels. The pulse-echo system is used to image the target blood vessel, and to guide the Doppler beam. The cross-sectional area and orientation of the blood vessel can be measured from the image and these, together with the Doppler shift signal, are used to estimate the volumetric flow. Potentially the technique is of tremendous value, but there are several errors inherent in the method which need to be appreciated if the best possible accuracy is to be achieved, and if realistic confidence limits are to be placed on such measurements.

The time averaged volumetric flow through a blood vessel, $\bar{Q}$, may be written:

$$\bar{Q} = \frac{1}{T} \int_{t=0}^{T} A(t)\, \bar{v}(t)\, dt \tag{1}$$

where $A(t)$ is the cross-sectional area of the vessel, and $\bar{v}(t)$ the instantaneous mean velocity. If the vessel is uniformly insonated by an ultrasound beam, then the instantaneous mean velocity may be estimated using the well known Doppler equation:

$$\bar{v}(t) = \frac{\bar{f}_d(t)\, c}{2 f_t \cos\theta} \tag{2}$$

where $\bar{f}_d(t)$ is the mean Doppler shift, c the velocity of ultrasound in blood, f_t the transmitted zero crossing frequency, and θ the angle between the ultrasound beam and the blood vessel. Substituting equation 2 into equation 1 allows the volumetric flow to be written in terms of the geometry of the vessel and the Doppler shift frequency:

$$\bar{Q} = \frac{c}{2 f_t \cos\theta} \int_{t=0}^{T} \frac{A(t)\, \bar{f}_d(t)\, dt}{T} \tag{3}$$

It is usual to assume that changes in vessel area over the cardiac cycle are insignificant, or at least cancel each other out, in which case equation 3 can be rewritten in a simplified form:

$$\bar{Q} = \frac{cA}{2f_t \cos\theta} \int_{t=0}^{T} \frac{\bar{f}_d(t)}{T} \, dt \qquad (4)$$

where A is the 'effective vessel area'. The zero crossing frequency of the transmitted signal is easily measured and the velocity of sound in blood is more or less constant, but each of the other terms in equation 4 ($\bar{f}_d$, A, and θ) is subject to measurement or interpretation errors which are discussed below.

19.2 Mean Doppler shift

The correct calculation of instantaneous mean velocity depends on the validity of equation 2, and the ability of the scanner to derive the true mean frequency of the Doppler spectrum. Necessary conditions for the validity of equation 2 are that the bandwidth of the transmitted signal is small compared with its centre frequency, and that scattered energy is received equally from all portions of the vessel cross-section. The former condition is usually met in duplex systems which rely on 'uniform insonation', but the latter is much more difficult to satisfy.

19.2.1 Transmitted signal bandwidth

Duplex scanners may incorporate either continuous wave (CW) or pulsed wave (PW) Doppler units and the relative merits of the two types of device are discussed elsewhere in this report[1]. The signal from a CW unit is monochromatic, but the bandwidth to centre frequency ratio (B_t/f_t) of the signal from a PW unit is influenced by the pulse length, and is approximately equal to the reciprocal of the number of oscillations in the transmitted burst. Both Rayleigh scattering and attenuation of ultrasound are frequency dependent and if B_t/f_t is large then these effects can significantly shift the centre frequency of a pulse from its transmitted value. This in turn will shift the mean Doppler frequency. Fortunately, if the whole of a vessel is to be within the sample volume, the sample gate of a PW unit must be wider than $2R/\sin\theta$, where R is the radius of the vessel, and therefore relatively long bursts of ultrasound with a low B_t/f_t are used. For this reason the finite transmitted signal bandwidth should not be a major source of inaccuracy in the measurement of blood flow velocity. Equations describing the effects of Rayleigh scattering and frequency dependent attenuation on the measured Doppler spectrum have been derived by Newhouse et al[2] and are summarised elsewhere in this report[1].

19.2.2 Uniform scattering

Equation 2 is only valid if scattered energy is received equally from the entire cross-section of the vessel. Scattering of ultrasound from blood is almost entirely due to erythrocytes[3], (or more strictly the local fluctuations in the concentration of the erythrocytes — see reference 1) which can be considered to be distributed uniformly in vessels with diameters of 1 mm or more where their size is negligible compared with that of the vessel[4]. Variations in scattered energy are therefore virtually entirely due to non-uniform illumination of the vessel by the incident ultrasound beam. This may be the result of the use of an ultrasound beam which is too narrow to sample the whole vessel uniformly, a result of shadowing by overlying structures, or the result of refraction and total reflection when the ultrasound beam strikes the vessel wall. Shadowing by overlying structures (such as by a calcified plaque) should be recognised in the B-mode image[5], and flow estimation not attempted, and for values of θ larger than 30°, less than 5 per cent of the vessel lumen is shadowed[5] and will cause a minimal error. The use of an ultrasound beam which is narrower than the vessel can however lead to larger errors.

The errors caused by partial sampling of the vessel may be calculated simply by considering the interaction between a weighting function $\zeta(r)$ and the time averaged mean component of the velocity profile $v_0(r)$[6]. The shape of $v_0(r)$ depends on many factors, and has different shapes in different parts of the body (see *reference 6* for a fuller discussion) but in general varies from being flat in the aortic arch to parabolic in the distal portion of vessels such as the femoral and carotid arteries. If $v_0(r)$ is flat then partial sampling of the vessel still produces a correct estimate of the mean velocity, but as the profile develops, then partial sampling will lead to progressively larger errors. A simple model[7], which assumes the ultrasound beam to be rectangular in cross-section, shows that the output of a mean frequency processor could overestimate the mean velocity by a factor of up to 33 per cent. Real ultrasound beams are not rectangular, and their shapes depend on factors such as whether the Doppler unit is PW or CW (in which case the transmitting and receiving crystals are separate), and the distance between the probe and vessel, but the results obtained using such a model show how important uniform insonation is. *Figure 19.1* shows the percentage error predicted by this model as a function of the ultrasonic beam width divided by the vessel diameter (τ). It can be seen that the error rises rapidly as τ decreases, suggesting that even small variations in the ultrasonic field strength across the vessel may lead to significant errors.

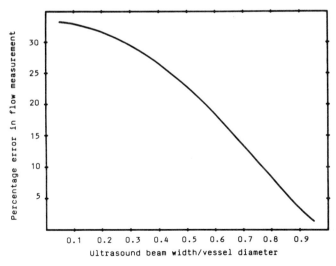

Figure 19.1 Percentage error in flow measurement due to partial insonation of a blood vessel containing flow whose time averaged velocity profile is parabolic.

147

19.2.3 Mean frequency processors

There are several approaches to the estimation of mean frequency from the Doppler spectrum. It may be implemented using a microprocessor linked to a spectrum analyser, or using the analogue circuits described by Arts and Roevros[8] or DeJong et al[9, 10]. The popular zero-crossing detector is not suitable in this application because its output is proportional to the root mean square of the input signal and not the mean frequency[11]. Similarly devices which calculate the modal frequency are to be avoided at least until such time as it is shown that their use does not introduce significant errors. Even true mean frequency processors are subject to errors which limit their accuracy, but these can to a certain extent be predicted and therefore corrected[12].

The Doppler signal returning from a target blood vessel inevitably contains a large clutter component at frequencies corresponding to low velocities. These signals result from several sources, notably movements of the vessel wall. The amplitude of these signals may be considerably greater than the blood flow signal, and they must therefore be rejected using high-pass filters. This also means that some of the wanted signals from low velocity blood flow are also rejected, and leads to an overestimation of the mean velocity. Gill[12] in a valuable discussion of mean frequency processor performance has shown that the error this produces depends on both the cut-off frequency of the filter f_{LP}, and the shape of the velocity profile, and can be estimated from:

$$\Delta f = \frac{2\,f_{LP}}{2+\beta} \tag{5}$$

where β is a factor which describes the velocity profile ($\beta = 2$ for parabolic flow and ∞ for plug flow). This could clearly lead to substantial errors if not allowed for; unfortunately the shape of the velocity profile changes throughout the cardiac cycle and this may therefore not always be possible.

The presence of interfering noise will also bias the output of a mean frequency processor and it has been shown by both Gerzberg and Meindl[13] and Gill[12] that this has the effect of (a) offsetting the frequency output by $f_n/(1+S)$, where f_n is the demodulator output that would be obtained with only the noise present, and S is the signal to noise ratio, and (b) reducing the slope of the demodulator output by a factor of $(1+1/S)$. These expressions could be used to correct for the effects of noise, but often the characteristics of the noise are not known and change from reading to reading. Further errors may be caused by double sideband generation in frequency offset systems, and by high Doppler frequency aliasing in pulsed Doppler systems. Gill[12] has shown that to cause an error of more than 1 per cent the spurious sideband (which appears as a mirror image of the Doppler spectrum and is due to imperfect circuit performance) must be less than 23 dB below the true sideband, and that under ideal circumstances where the spurious sideband is 35–40 dB down, the error is of the order of 0.05 per cent. High frequency aliasing occurs when the pulse repetition frequency (PRF) of a PW Doppler unit is less than twice the highest Doppler shift present, and should be avoided either by the use of a sufficiently high PRF, or CW Doppler.

19.3 Vessel area

Volumetric flow is proportional to vessel area and therefore an error in measuring the area is directly reflected as a similar error in flow measurement. The vessel area changes during the cardiac cycle, and thus the correct way to calculate flow is to integrate the vessel area — instantaneous mean Doppler shift product over the cardiac cycle. Commercial duplex scanners presently available do not have this facility, and the area of the vessel must therefore be measured independently from the mean Doppler shift. There are therefore two components to the vessel area error, that due to the limited accuracy of equation 4, and that due to difficulties in measuring any area accurately.

19.3.1 Changes during the cardiac cycle

A number of methods of monitoring changes in the arterial diameter during the cardiac cycle have been described[14-17], but to date surprisingly few studies of these changes have been reported, and the majority deal with either the fetal aorta or the adult common carotid artery. Hokanson et al[14] reported changes of approximately 1 mm in the diameter of the adult femoral artery, which is equivalent to about 14 per cent, whilst values of between 5 per cent and 10 per cent have been reported for the adult common carotid artery[18, 19], and between 10 per cent and 17 per cent for the fetal aorta[20, 21]. These changes cannot be ignored in flow measurements, especially as a 10 per cent diameter change in a cylindrical vessel is approximately equivalent to a 20 per cent area change. Most duplex scanners calculate flow using a single diameter or area taken at random, and this can lead to large and unpredictable errors. Short of evaluating the vessel area — instantaneous mean Doppler shift integral, there is no way to completely eliminate this error, but it may be reduced by measuring the vessel diameter on a number of occasions and using the mean or median vessel diameter in the flow calculation. Struyk et al[21] investigated the accuracy of flow measurements made in the descending aortas of fetal lambs, and found that the use of the maximum diameter of the vessel led to a mean error of +9.1 per cent, and that use of the minimum diameter produced a mean error of −18.6 per cent. Use of the mean of the maximum and minimum diameters $(D_{max}+D_{min})/2$, and the time averaged diameter gave errors of −4.8 per cent and −5.4 per cent respectively. It may be possible to correct measurements in the fetus for a known systematic error, but it is unlikely that a simple correction will be possible in adults with vascular disease where the disease process interferes with vessel compliance and changes in vessel dimensions.

19.3.2 Measurement of diameter

It is possible to measure the cross-sectional area of a vessel directly (see next section), but it is more usual to measure its diameter, and to calculate the area by assuming it to be cylindrical. Most normal arteries are approximately circular in cross-section, but this is not true of veins, and of arteries with arteriosclerotic involvement, where the disease process may affect one aspect of the vessel more than others[22]. It is therefore important to examine the cross-sectional image of a vessel before making diameter measurements, to ensure that the vessel is at least roughly circular in cross-section.

Measurement of the vessel diameter itself is also open to errors, primarily due to the limited resolution achievable using ultrasound. A particular problem is that because of the limited axial resolution, echoes from the inner and outer surfaces of a blood vessel (and perhaps even the different layers within the wall) tend to merge together and therefore only the first echo is reliable. Because of this, workers in the field of fetal blood flow have tended to measure from the outer

149

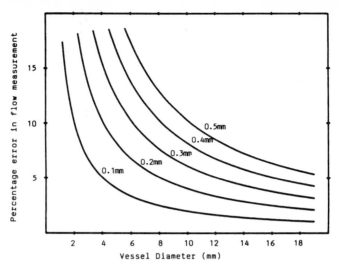

Figure 19.2 Percentage error in flow measurement due to the uncertainty in the diameter measurement (± 0.1 mm to ± 0.5 mm) plotted as a function of diameter.

aspect of the proximal wall to the inner aspect of the distal wall[20, 23]. This produces an overestimate which could be reduced if the thickness of the wall of the vessel were known. At best it seems, because of the unpredictable phase changes which occur at interfaces, that the obtainable accuracy is of the order of a wavelength of the imaging ultrasound. *Figure 19.2* shows the percentage error in measured flow plotted against vessel diameter for various errors in that measurement. Keeping in mind that the wavelength of ultrasound with frequencies of 3 MHz, 5 MHz, and 10 MHz are 0.5 mm, 0.3 mm, and 0.15 mm respectively, it can be seen that potential errors in measurements on vessels of less than 5 mm diameter can be very high indeed.

One further error, which can be allowed for, is that due to the difference in the velocity of ultrasound in 'soft-tissues' and blood. The calipers of most B-scanners are set to around 1540 m s^{-1}, whilst the velocity of ultrasound in blood is about 1580 m s^{-1}. This will lead to an underestimate of the vessel diameter by 2.6 per cent (and of flow by 5.2 per cent) unless steps are taken to correct for it. As pointed out by Eik-Nes *et al*[20] this tends to compensate for the error introduced by measuring the vessel diameter from the outer to inner aspect of the vessel.

19.3.3 Measurement of area

The direct measurement of the vessel area by rotating the scan head 90° around the vertical axis to produce a cross-sectional view of the vessel seems at first sight an attractive alternative to diameter measurement, since it means that no assumptions need be made about the shape of the vessel. This technique has, however, two drawbacks which have discouraged its use. The first is that once the probe is shifted it is very difficult to ensure that the cross-sectional area being measured is at the same point at which the velocity was measured. This is particulary difficult if the Doppler transducer is built into the same head as the

150

imaging transducer, since the Doppler signal is unlikely to be obtained from the vessel directly below the probe, expecially if the vessel runs roughly parallel to the skin surface. The second problem is that the lateral resolution of pulse-echo imaging transducers is not as good as the axial resolution, and furthermore it is difficult to obtain a good image of the edges of a circular target because their orientation leads to a small degree of back-scatter. Thus the apparent advantages of imaging the whole cross-section may be outweighed by the difficulties of locating the correct cross-section, and even then of making accurate measurements.

19.4   Angle of insonation

The final variable in equation 4 which needs to be measured is the angle θ between the ultrasound beam and the blood vessel. Since it is the cosine of θ which determines the component of velocity which is measured by the Doppler probe, the error introduced by a given uncertainty in θ ($\delta\theta$) is a function of θ itself, and increases rapidly with θ. The percentage error in flow measurement is plotted as a function of θ for several values of $\delta\theta$ in *figure 19.3*. With care it should be possible to measure θ to $\pm2°$ or under ideal conditions to $\pm1°$ (although some scanners do not have this resolution in their angle measuring cursor), and thus provided θ itself is kept below 60°, and preferably below 45°, the error in flow measurement should not be excessive. It is worth noting that keeping θ below 45° is much easier if the Doppler probe is mounted separately from the imaging probe.

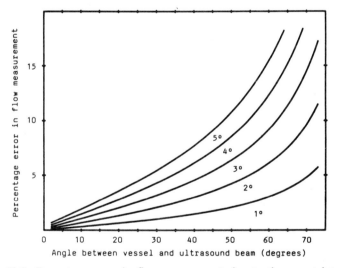

Figure 19.3   Percentage error in flow measurement due to the uncertainty in the measurement of the angle ($\pm1°$ to $\pm5°$) between the ultrasound beam and the axis of the blood vessel, plotted as a function of angle.

19.5   Discussion and conclusions

There are numerous sources of error in volumetric blood-flow measurements made using a duplex scanner. Many of them can be virtually eliminated by careful technique, but some are difficult to control. *Table 19.1* summarises what should be the major sources of error if reasonable precautions are taken. The magnitudes of these errors are to a certain extent dictated by the vessel in which the measurement is to be made, but the scanner itself can influence them.

Measurement of mean velocity depends on uniform insonation of the vessel, which is easier to achieve in vessels of small diameter, but the converse is true with diameter measurement, and it is difficult to see how, using current techniques, volumetric flow measurements can be made in vessels of less than about 4 or 5 mm in diameter. Most commercial scanners rely on a single diameter from which to estimate area, and this is clearly unsatisfactory in vessels which are pulsating, and users should be encouraged to make a number of determinations of the diameter before arriving at a final figure. It is important to keep the angle θ as low as possible, and certainly below 60°, if the error due to angle measurement is not to become significant, and this is much easier using duplex heads which have a separate off-set Doppler probe. This arrangement is also advantageous where the operator wishes to measure vessel area directly, since the Doppler probe can be aimed at the vessel directly below the centre of the imaging head, thus facilitating the measurement of the correct data.

Table 19.1 Summary of major sources of error.

Source	Comments and typical values for errors
Non-uniform ultrasound beam	Depends on time averaged velocity profile and relative size of ultrasound beam and vessel. The error is negligible if there is plug flow, but may be of the order of $+30\%$ if a narrow beam is used to interrogate parabolic flow. See *figure 19.1*
High-pass filters (to eliminate vessel wall thump etc.)	$\Delta f \simeq 2 \, f_{LP}/(2 + \beta)$ (See text for explanation of symbols)
Vessel pulsatility	Depends on vessel elasticity, flow pulsatility, and the way in which the vessel diameter is measured, For single random measurements the flow error may vary between -20% and $+10\%$; use of an average of ten measurements may reduce this to between 0 and -5%.
Diameter measurement	Depends on the frequency of the imaging ultrasound and on the size of the vessel. Typical minimum flow errors for vessels of 4 mm, 6 mm, and 8 mm might be $\pm15\%$, $\pm10\%$, and $\pm8\%$. See *figure 19.2*
Vessel shape	Calculation of area from a single diameter assumes a circular vessel cross-section. This may be a major source of error in veins and diseased arteries.
Angle measurement	Depends on the value of the angle to be measured. Typical flow errors for angles of 15°, 30°, 45°, and 60° might be $<1\%$, 1–2%, 2–3%, and 3–5%. See *figure 19.3*.
Miscellaneous	Several of the other errors discussed in the text may become highly significant if great care is not taken to minimise them.

It is important to distinguish between systematic and random errors, since the former will not greatly influence studies on change of flow, and may even be standardised between patients and different centres. Examples of these are the error due to the use of a given high pass filter, those due to measuring the vessel diameter from the outer to inner aspect of the walls, and those due to an incorrect velocity setting for the calipers. Random errors on the other hand will affect even the intra-subject error and must be monitored carefully. These include that due to vessel pulsations, measurement of the diameter (once the technique has been settled) and the measurement of the angle θ. Some random errors may be reduced by repeated measurement of the same parameter, but this is not always so.

There is no simple answer as to whether duplex scanners can measure volumetric flow. There are sites from which flow measurements must be regarded as impossible, but equally there are sites from which measurements may be made with sufficient accuracy to be of clinical use. The magnitude of possible errors must be carefully considered before the values obtained using a duplex scanner are treated as reliable. It is worth noting that equation 2 which is an expression for mean velocity, can be much more accurately evaluated than equation 3, and that there are many circumstances in which mean velocity may be as valuable as mean flow.

References

1   EVANS D H 1986 Doppler ultrasound signals from blood flow In *Physics in Medical Ultrasound* (Ed. J A Evans) Chapter 15 (IPSM, 47 Belgrave Square, London)
2   NEWHOUSE V L, EHRENWALD A R and JOHNSON G F 1977 The effect of Rayleigh scattering and frequency dependent absorption on the output spectrum of Doppler blood flowmeters In *Ultrasound in Medicine* **3B** (Eds D White and R E Brown) 1181–1191 (Plenum press, New York)
3   SHUNG K K, SIGELMANN R A and REID J M 1976 Scattering of ultrasound by blood *IEEE Trans Biomed Engng* **BME—23** 460–467
4   McDONALD D A 1974 *Blood flow in arteries* pp 55–70 (Arnold, London)
5   GILL R W 1982 Accuracy calculations for ultrasonic pulsed Doppler blood flow measurements *Australasian Physical and Engng Sci in Med* **5** 51–57
6   EVANS D H 1985 On the measurement of the mean velocity of blood flow over the cardiac cycle using Doppler ultrasound *Ultrasound Med Biol* **11** 735–741
7   EVANS D H 1982 Some aspects of the relationship between instantaneous volumetric blood flow and continuous wave Doppler ultrasound recordings–I. The effect of ultrasonic beam width on the output of maximum, mean and rms frequency processors *Ultrasound Med Biol* **6** 605–609
8   ARTS M G J and ROEVROS J M J G 1972 On the instantaneous measurement of bloodflow by ultrasonic means *Med Biol Engng* **10** 23–34
9   DeJONG D A, MEGENS P H A, DeVLIEGER M, THON H and HOLLAND W P J 1975 A direction quantifying Doppler system for measurement of transport velocity of blood *Ultrasonics* **13** 138–141
10   GERZBERG L and MEINDL J D 1980 The root f power-spectrum centroid detector: System considerations, implementation, and performance *Ultrasonic Imaging* **2** 262–289
11   RICE S O 1944 Mathematical analysis of random noise *Bell Syst Tech J* **23** 282–332
12   GILL R W 1979 Performance of the mean frequency Doppler modulator *Ultrasound Med Biol* **5** 237–247
13   GERZBERG L and MEINDL J D 1977 Mean frequency estimator with applications in ultrasonic Doppler flowmeters In *Ultrasound in Medicine* **3B** (Ed D White and R E Brown) 1173–1180 (Plenum press, New York)

14 HOKANSON D E, STRANDNESS D E and MILLER W C 1970 An echo tracking system for recording arterial wall motion *IEEE Trans Sonics Ultrason* **SU–17** 130–132

15 OLSEN C F 1977 Doppler ultrasound: A technique for obtaining arterial wall motion parameters *IEEE Trans Sonics Ultrason* **SU–24** 354–358

16 GROVES D H, POWALOWSKI T and WHITE D N 1982 A digital technique for tracking moving interfaces *Ultrasound Med Biol* **8** 185–190

17 HOEKS A P G, RUISSEN C J, HICK P and RENEMAN R S 1985 Transcutaneous detection of relative changes in artery diameter *Ultrasound Med Biol* **11** 51–59

18 RENEMAN R S, VAN MERODE T, HOEKS A P G and HICK P The on-line recording of velocity profiles and diameter changes in normal and stenosed cervical carotid arteries in man (Abstract) *Ultrasound Med Biol* **8** Suppl 1 161

19 UEMATSU S, YANG A, PREZIOSI T J, KOUBA R and TOUNG J K 1983 Measurement of carotid blood flow in man and its clinical application *Stroke* **14** 256–266

20 EIK-NES S H, MARSAL K, BRUBAKK A O, KRISTOFFERSON K and ULSTEIN M 1982 Ultrasonic measurement of human fetal blood flow *J Biomed Engng* **4** 28–36

21 STRUYK P C, PIJPERS L, WLADIMIROFF J W, LOTGERING F K, TONGE M and BOM N 1985 The time-distance recorder as a means of improving the accuracy of fetal blood flow measurements *Ultrasound Med Biol* **11** 71–77

22 STEPHENSON S E, MANN G V, YOUNGER R and SCOTT H W 1962 Factors influencing the segmental deposition of atheromatous material *Arch Surg* **84** 49–55

23 TEAGUE M J, WILLSON K, BATTYE C K, TAYLOR M G, GRIFFIN D R, CAMPBELL S and ROBERTS V C 1985 A combined ultrasonic linear array scanner and pulsed Doppler velocimeter for the estimation of blood flow in the fetus and adult abdomen—I: Technical aspects *Ultrasound Med Biol* **11** 27–36

CHAPTER 20

Measurements of Maximum Velocity using CW Ultrasound

W F Tait
University Department of Surgery, Withington Hospital, Manchester M20

20.1 Introduction

Atherosclerotic disease of the carotid bifurcation is important as a cause of stroke. As medical or surgical treatment is available the accurate identification of disease at this site is essential. Although ulceration without narrowing may occur in the early stages of the disease, as the disease progresses a stenosis develops. The presence of a stenosis is important haemodynamically as it causes the velocity of flow in the artery to increase as it goes through the stenosis. The use of Doppler shifted ultrasound to record velocities is a well established technique and the maximum frequency (ΔF_{max}) at peak systole measured by continuous wave (CW) ultrasound is often used to grade stenoses. However ΔF_{max} is affected by the angle of insonation (θ) which can only be estimated using standard techniques. We devised a method to measure θ and calculate the maximum velocity (V_{max}) at peak systole which might allow more reliable measurements to be made in patients.

20.2 Theory

The method involved taking two measurements of ΔF_{max} from the same arterial sampling site using a single transducer when the angle (W) between the two measurements is known. In practice we have used an angle of 10°. The theory was derived from the Doppler formula and when W equals 10°

$$\tan \theta = \left(\cos 10° - \frac{\Delta F_{max\,1}}{\Delta F_{max\,2}} \right) \cdot \frac{1}{\sin 10°}$$

Once θ was known it was simple to convert a measurement of ΔF_{max} into one of V_{max} using the Doppler formula.

20.3 Experiment

Having devised a method from theory the limits of its practical application were investigated. Hence the relationship between ΔF_{max} and θ was studied both in a laboratory model and in patients. With the velocity of flow constant in a model a linear relationship between ΔF_{max} and $\cos \theta$ was anticipated for values of θ between 0° and 90°. The first experiment to investigate the relationship between ΔF_{max} and θ was carried out in a model. An emulsion of milk was circulated through a circuit of tubing and ultrasound recordings were taken from the test section with the angle of insonation of the ultrasound probe varied between 0° and 90°. Signals were recorded using the 4 MHz probe of a CW ultrasound instrument. It was found that ΔF_{max} increased as θ decreased from 90° until a critical angle of 40° was reached whereupon ΔF_{max} decreased. There was a linear relationship between ΔF_{max} and $\cos \theta$ but only for values of $\theta > 40°$. At $\theta = 90°$ ΔF_{max} should theoretically be zero but that it is not, is explained by the arrangement of the crystals in the transducer and the divergence of the ultrasound beam. The explanation for the decrease in ΔF_{max} below the critical angle of 40° was not apparent and further experiments showed that it was not due to the ultrasound reflector in the medium, the coupling agent between probe and tube, or the ultrasound instrument and level of gain. Moreover, the phenomenon occurred under conditions of both steady and oscillatory flow.

A hypothesis that the ultrasound beam was being reflected from the surface of the tubing once θ was less than the critical angle, and furthermore that from the laws of refraction this critical angle should vary with the material or tubing, was investigated in the model. For this purpose a hydrophone was used which could detect high frequency sound waves up to the order of approximately 10 MHz. The hydrophone, ultrasound probe and tubing to be tested were arranged in a water tank and as the probe was rotated between 0° and 90° to the tubing, so too was the hydrophone to give an equal angle of incidence with the tubing. The hydrophone was connected to an oscilloscope and it was found that once the ultrasound probe was below the critical angle a sudden increase in signal from the hydrophone was recorded. This was due to a total reflection of the ultrasound beam from the surface of the tube. Tubing of different materials was tested and the critical angles for Goretex (a vascular prosthesis manufactured from PTFE) was 51°, calcified artery 25° and normal artery 15°.

20.4   Patient studies

Having explained the decrease in ΔF_{max} for values of θ less than the critical angle, the relationships between them was explored in the common carotid arteries of 8 patients. Multiple ultrasound signals were recorded between 0° and 180° in intervals of 10° from the same site in the carotid artery using a protractor attached to the ultrasound probe. The signals were recorded using a CW Doppler imaging system. The lowest value of ΔF_{max} was assumed to be when θ was 90° and other values of θ could then be calculated as there was 10° between measurements. Once a critical angle was reached three varieties of response were found:

(i) ΔF_{max} decreased
(ii) No ultrasound signal could be detected
(iii) A plateau response, i.e. ΔF_{max} stayed at the same level until no ultrasound signal could be detected.

The critical angle in 16 carotid arteries was calculated from the mean of all these responses and was approximately 30°. Again there was a linear relationship between ΔF_{max} and $\cos \theta$ but only between 30° and 80°.

20.5   Conclusions

These experiments showed that the method of measuring θ could be expected to work for values of θ between 30° and 80° in patients. We used a protractor attached to the spatial sensing arm of a Doppler imaging system to measure the angle W and found it to be a simple but efficient method of calculating V_{max}. When one insonates the carotid artery blindly and presumes that the optimum signal is at 60° or 45° there is a considerable margin of error which can be avoided by determining the true velocity. We believe our method is an improvement over other methods of calculating the angle of insonation and maximum velocity.

156

CHAPTER 21

Extension of the KLM Transducer Model to Doppler Probes

D Follett and D Peake
Medical Physics Department, Bristol General Hospital, 1–2 Redcliffe Parade West, Bristol BS1 6SP

21.1 Introduction

The KLM model of the ultrasound transducer[1] has been used for some time now to predict the behaviour of transducers under different conditions of electrical and acoustic load. Pulse echo transducers require relatively heavy external damping to achieve an adequately wide bandwidth. The external damping is achieved either by adding a lossy medium, e.g. epoxy resin impregnated with tungsten powder, to the back face of the transducer, or, by coupling the transducer more effectively to the load by means of one or more quarter-wave matching layers. For such transducers predicted and measured behaviour agree well.

When the KLM model is applied to lightly damped PZT transducers the calculated and measured values of the electrical input impedance are found to be grossly in error. This situation requires the introduction of an attenuation constant in the acoustic transmission line equations as mentioned by Silk[2] to represent losses in the transducer material. This paper presents some preliminary results showing the improvement in the prediction of electrical input impedance and acoustic output for lightly loaded transducers such as therapy and Doppler probes when such damping is incorporated in the KLM model.

The required attenuation constant was found for the ferroelectric ceramics PZT5A, PZT5H and PZT4 for frequencies in the range 1 to 10 MHz. Where reference is made to the transducer under test in this report it refers to a disc of PZT5H of resonant frequency 2.6 MHz and 5 mm in diameter. The graphs and tables presented in this report also refer to the same PZT5H transducer unless otherwise stated.

21.2 The KLM model

Before discussing the KLM model, which includes an acoustic transmission line, a brief treatment of the theory of transmission lines is given for completeness.

A lossless transmission line is completely characterised by its characteristic impendance Z_0 and wave velocity c. For a wave of frequency f the phase constant β is given by

$$\beta = \frac{2\pi f}{c} \text{ radians/unit length} \tag{1}$$

For a lossy line, in the electrical case if the voltage decays from V_0 to V_χ over distance χ then the decay constant α is given by

$$\alpha = \frac{1}{\chi} \log_e \frac{V_o}{V_x} \text{ Nepers/unit length} \tag{2}$$

(1 Neper = 8.686 dB)

If a transmission line of length d is loaded with an impedance $Z_L = R_L + j\,X_L$ at its far end, the input impendance Z_1 is given by the standard transmission line equation

$$Z_1 = Z_o \left[\frac{(R_L + j\,X_L) \cosh(\alpha + j\beta)d + Z_o \sinh(\alpha + j\beta)d}{Z_o \cosh(\alpha + j\beta)d + (R_L + j\,X_L) \sinh(\alpha + j\beta)d} \right] \tag{3}$$

Also the voltage V_L appearing across the load due to an input voltage of V_1 is given by

$$V_L = V_1 \left[\frac{R_L + j\,X_L}{(R_L + j\,X_L) \cosh(\alpha + j\beta)d + Z_o \sinh(\alpha + j\beta)d} \right] \tag{4}$$

Figure 21.1 shows the complete equivalent circuit of the plate transducer operating in its thickness mode and *table 21.1* defines the components used in the equivalent circuit as well as giving the values of the parameters used for the transducer under test. The excitation electrical voltage Vs is transformed into an acoustic force at the centre of an acoustic transmission line. For the MKS system of units:

1 volt represents a force of 1 Newton
1 amp represents a particle velocity of 1 ms^{-1}

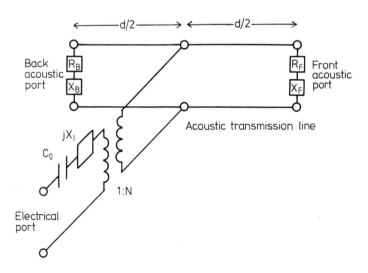

Figure 21.1   The KLM model of an ultrasound transducer. See *table 21.1* for the definition of the parameters d, Co, jX$_1$ and N.

Table 21.1 KLM equivalent circuit components.

Parameter	Meaning	Parameter value for PZT 5H transducer
C_0	$A\epsilon^s_{33}/d$	
A	area of plate	20 mm²
ρ	density of plate	7.500 kg m⁻³
c	speed of sound in plate	4560 ms⁻¹
Z_T	$A\rho c$	
d	thickness	0.77 mm
f	frequency	
$\epsilon^s_{33}/\epsilon_0$	relative dielectric constant, clamped	1470
ϵ_0	dielectric constant of free space	8.85 × 10⁻¹² Fm⁻¹
h_{33}	piezoelectric constant	18 × 10⁸ Vm⁻¹
X_1	$Z_T M^2 \sin(2\pi fd/c)$	
N	$(1/2M) \operatorname{cosec}(\pi fd/c)$	
M	$h_{33}/2\pi f Z_T$	

$R_F + jX_F$ and $R_B + jX_B$ represent the acoustic impedances at the front and back surfaces respectively. The characteristic impedance per unit area, Z_0, is given by ρc, hence for a transducer of cross sectional area A the characteristic impedance Z_T is given by $\rho c A$. The characteristic impedance of water Z_w is taken as 1.48×10^6 kg m⁻² s⁻¹ (Rayl).

To find the electrical input impedance of the transducer the back and front loads of the transducer are reflected to the centre of the transmission line using equation 3, these are added in parallel and then reflected across the electroacoustic transformer. To find the force at the surface of the transducer the acoustic force at the centre of the transmission line is found for a given electrical input voltage and then using equation 4, the force at the front and back faces can be calculated.

At the fundamental undamped resonant frequency of the transducer the transmission line is a half wavelength long, the next active harmonic occurring theoretically at three times the fundamental frequency.

21.3 Measurements and results

21.3.1 Transducer input impedance

The electrical input impedance of each transducer was found using an Hewlett Packard 4193A vector impedance meter which gives the impedance in the form $Z\,|\underline{\theta}$. Alternative representation of the input impedances are (a) series resistance and capacitance, and (b) parallel resistance (RP) and capacitance (CP), where a negative capacitance in (a) and (b) represents inductance.

The parallel resistance and capacitance representation has been adopted as it was felt that this gave an intuitive feel of how the acoustic pressure output changed with frequency.

Since electrical power into the transducer is proportional to $(RP)^{-1}$ and acoustic pressure is proportional to (acoustic power)$^{1/2}$, it follows that the acoustic output pressure is proportional to $(RP)^{-1/2}$.

The parallel equivalent is also generally more useful for designing electrical matching and timing networks. *Figures 21.2a and 21.2b* show the measured

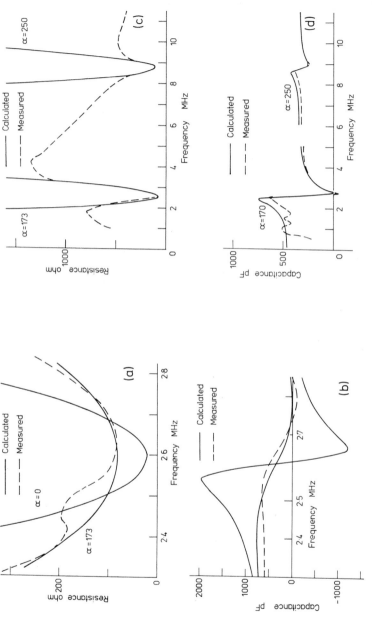

Figure 21.2 Calculated and measured frequency response of the PZT 5H transducer of, (a) the equivalent parallel input resistance (b) the equivalent parallel input capacitance, showing the effect of including an acoustic attenuation constant, α, in the calculations. (c) and (d) show that a larger attenuation constant at the higher resonant frequency is required for good agreement between calculated and measured values.

160

frequency response of RP and CP for the transducer under test with values predicted by the KLM model with and without the inclusion of a transmission line attenuation constant. *Figures 21.2c and 21.2d* show the results including the attenuation constant on an extended frequency scale to include the third harmonic response. Note that for the third harmonic part a different attenuation constant was used to obtain agreement with the measured results.

Figure 21.3 shows the normalised theoretical and measured frequency responses of the pressure at the front surface of the transducer and $RP^{-1/2}$. The next section explains how the pressure at the front face of the transducer was measured. The frequency response of the acoustic output pressure assumes a constant electrical excitation voltage.

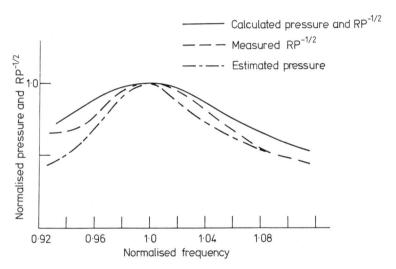

Figure 21.3 The normalised frequency response of the measured and calculated values of the acoustic pressure at the front face of the transducer and the reciprocal of the square root of the equivalent parallel input resistance, RP.

21.3.2 Acoustic output pressure

A calibrated Marconi PVDF bilaminar membrane hydrophone was used to detect the acoustic pressure radially to the beam's central axis at a distance of 5 cm from the transducer's front face, i e. in the Fraunhofer region, to obtain a pressure profile. If the beam is radially symmetrical its cross-section can be divided into n annual rings, for the ith of which the area is a_i and the pressure P_i. The total power in the beam is proportional to $\sum_{1}^{n} a_i P_i^2$.

To find the pressure at the front face of the transducer it is assumed that it behaves as an oscillating piston of area A and pressure P_t, with the power radiating from it proportional to AP_t^2. It follows that

$$P_t = \left(\frac{K \sum_{1}^{n} a_i P_i^2}{A} \right)^{1/2} \tag{5}$$

where K is a correction factor for the attenuation between the transducer and the hydrophone.

Transmission loss is defined as:

$$10 \log_e \frac{\text{Electrical power input}}{\text{Acoustic power output}}$$

In *table 21.2* the first three rows of data compare the measured values of the minimum value of RP (which occurs at 2.6 MHz) and the transmission loss for the air backed transducer, with the calculated values for no internal damping and with the attenuation constant that gives the best agreement with the measured RP. It will be seen that with no internal damping the calculated figures are greatly in

Table 21.2 Values of RP and transmission loss at 2.6 MHz for different backing layer characteristic impedances. Transducer is loaded with water.

	Z_0 of Backing layer	Transducer attenuation constant	Equivalent parallel resistance	Transmission loss
	Rayl	Nepers m^{-1}	ohms	dB
Measured values	3.3×10^{-4} (Air)	—	81	6.06
Calculated values	3.3×10^{-4} (Air)	0	20	0
	3.3×10^{-4}	173	81	6.13
	5	0	87	6.44
	5	173	147	8.73
	15	0	222	10.43
	15	173	277	11.44
	25	0	355	12.46
	25	173	399	13

Table 21.3 Calculated values of RP and transmission loss at 2.6 MHz for different quarter-wave matching layer characteristic impedances. Transducer is air backed and loaded with water.

Z_0 of matching layer	Transducer attenuation constant	Equivalent parallel resistance	Transmission loss
Rayl	Nepers m^{-1}	ohms	dB
None	0	20	0
None	173	81	6.13
2.66	0	65	0
2.66	173	125	2.98
4.215	0	162	0
4.215	173	219	1.53
7.11	0	462	0
7.11	173	492	0.87

error. The rest of *table 21.2* lists calculated values, without and with internal damping, for increasing backing layer damping. *Table 21.3* extends this for air backing but with a quarter-wave matching layer now providing increased external damping. As expected, the effect of internal losses becomes less important as external damping increases. However, *table 21.2* shows significant differences, particularly for RP, at values of backing layer impedance likely to be achieved in practice. In *table 21.2* the matching layer is assumed to be lossless; the values of Z_0 chosen are 2.66 for epoxy resin, 4.215 for optimally flat frequency response and 7.11 for optimum matching at the resonant frequency.

21.3.3   Transducer material attenuation constant

In most applications of the KLM model the attenuation constant of the transducer material is assumed to be zero which is only valid when the transducer is heavily damped.

In this study the attenuation constant was chosen so that, with the transducer air backed and loaded with water at its front surface, the measured and theoretical values of the minimum value of RP were the same. To extend the data for other materials and frequencies, the same criteria was used to find the attenuation constant for a number of other transducers, the results being shown in *figure 21.4* for three types of PZT ceramic. This figure should only be used to give an indication of the order of magnitude of the attenuation constant since only one transducer of each type was tested for a given frequency, and also the attenuation constant seems to be dependant upon the area of the transducer, an effect that was not investigated in detail in the present study. The 1 MHz transducers tested were all nominally 10 mm diameter, the rest were all nominally 5 mm diameter.

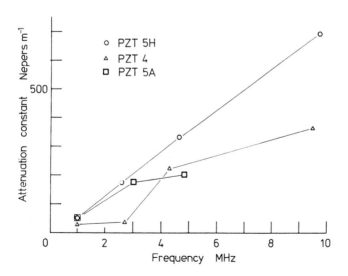

Figure 21.4   Measured values of acoustic attenuation for three types of PZT piezoelectric ceramic.

21.4 Discussion

From *figure 21.2* it can be seen that the first harmonic frequency of the transducer is 3.35 f_o (where f_o is the measured fundamental frequency) and not 3 f_o as predicted by simple theory; similar observations were made with other transducers. *Figure 21.2* also shows that a higher attenuation constant, 250 Nepers m^{-1}, is required for the measured and theoretical values of electrical input impedance to agree more closely at the third harmonic. Good agreement between the measured and calculated values of transmission loss was also found at the third harmonic frequency when the attenuation constant of 250 Nepers m^{-1} was used.

For all the transducers tested the theoretical frequencies at which the minimum values of RP occurred are lower than the measured value by between 1 and 8 per cent. For a given transducer the thickness across its faces was found to vary by up to 10 per cent; this, coupled with the possibility of the transducer's mechanical and piezoelectric properties not agreeing with the values given in the manufacturer's data sheets could introduce errors into the calculations.

It is also clear from *figure 21.2c* that even the modified model does not predict behaviour accurately except near the resonant frequencies, so it cannot be regarded as a true representation of a transducer. Nevertheless, the inclusion of an attenuation constant in the acoustic transmission line of the KLM model would seem a useful means for obtaining a more accurate prediction of the transducer's performance, particularly for transducers with light to medium damping.

References

1 KRIMHOLTZ R, LEEDOM D A and MATTAEI G L 1970 New equivalent circuits for elementary piezoelectric transducers *Electron Lett* **6** 398–399
2 SILK M G 1983 Predictions of the effect of some constructional variables on the performance of ultrasonic transducers *Ultrasonics* **21** 27–33

CHAPTER 22

Real-Time Scanners: Tissue Characterisation or Machine Characterisation?

R J Marsh, J E Gardner and G Cusick
Department of Medical Physics and Bioengineering, University College Hospital, 1st Floor–Shropshire House, 11–20 Capper Street, London WC1E 6JA

22.1 Introduction

It is over 30 years since the first measurement of the ultrasonic attenuation of tissue. Since then many techniques have been developed for estimating attenuation from both transmitted and backscattered radio frequency (RF) signals. Results obtained during this time have shown that attenuation, and its frequency dependence, vary with tissue pathology and structure[1]. If attenuation could be estimated precisely and conveniently in a clinical environment, it would provide a useful diagnostic tool, and would have applications in many fields, including the diagnosis of liver conditions[2], and the assessment of fetal lung maturity[3,4].

There are two main requirements in order to be able to use attenuation in clinical studies. The technique must have the precision to distinguish between pathological and normal tissue attenuation values for homogeneous samples, and it must be able to localise interrogated regions of homogeneous tissue within the subject. Even in extended tissues such as liver, precision should be improved by carefully selecting the interrogated region to be free of vessels and other inhomogeneities.

We set out to investigate the possibility of developing a clinically useful system for estimating attenuation in fetal lung. A commercial real-time scanner with a linear array transducer was modified for this purpose. The modifications enabled backscattered RF data to be digitised externally and stored on magnetic disc. An attenuation coefficient is estimated from this data using a spectral difference technique. The advantages of this system are that the organ, or area, of interest can be precisely located, and that the RF signal backscattered from that organ can be recorded while normal imaging is taking place. Whilst the static B-scanner is expected to produce better attenuation measurements, precise selection of the interrogated tissue is difficult or impossible as a result of tissue movement.

This paper describes investigations of the precision of the linear-array system for determining attenuation in a homogeneous medium provided by a commercially available tissue-equivalent phantom. Comparison is made with measurements performed using a single disc transducer attached to a static B-scanner.

22.2 Data analysis

The attenuation of soft tissue increases approximately linearly with frequency. Over small bandwidths (1–2 MHz) the relationship can be assumed to be linear. The slope of the attenuation vs frequency curve, denoted by β, has been shown to be an indicator of tissue state[5]. A number of methods for estimating β from backscattered signals have been proposed. Here, a version of the Spectral Difference technique is used. It is described by Kuc and Schwartz[2], and has been evaluated against other methods by Kuc[6]. The technique is illustrated in *figure 22.1*.

A line of RF data, or A-scan, is divided into two segments of equal length, a near segment and a far segment with respect to the transducer. Each segment is isolated using a Hamming window and its log power spectrum calculated. The Hamming window reduces sidelobes in the power spectra. The far spectrum is subtracted from the near spectrum, resulting in a curve of attenuation vs frequency. The slope of this curve, within the bandwidth of the transducer, is estimated using a least squares fit. The slope, divided by the distance between the centres of the segments, gives β in units of dB MHz^{-1} cm^{-1}.

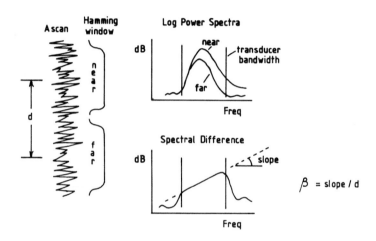

Figure 22.1   Estimation of β by the Log Spectral Difference Technique.

It should be noted that this is a statistical estimation. Due to the stochastic nature of scattering any one A-scan will only contain a sample of the spectral content of the interrogating pulse. This technique rests on the assumption that the scattering is random i.e. averaging over sufficient number of different A-scans will estimate the interrogating pulse for the near and far segments. The averaging is done after calculating the log power spectrum for each section.

22.3   Data acquisition system

Figure 22.2 is a block diagram of the system. An Hitachi EUB 25 real-time scanner, with a 3.5 MHz linear array transducer, has been modified so that an RF signal is available at a socket on the back panel. The RF signal is extracted as early as possible in the signal processing chain; although this is after amplification, bandpass filtering and time gain compensation (tgc). The RF signal is connected directly to a Biomation 8100 programmable transient recorder, which has a resolution of eight bits.

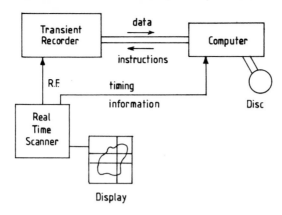

Display

Figure 22.2 Block diagram of the data collection system.

A second modification to the scanner enables a cursor, consisting of one vertical line and two horizontal lines, to be superimposed on the real-time ultrasound image. The cursor defines the sample region and can be moved about the screen by means of a small keypad so that a section of a vertical line in the image can be selected for recording. The timing and gating information, required to select this section from the continuous RF signal, is input to the computer. The computer programs the transient recorder with sampling rate, length of data segment and timing information. The operator has a sample button which triggers the collection of the RF data. The RF signal relating to the selected portion of the image is digitised, transmitted to the computer and stored on magnetic disc. Normally a number of these lines of data, or A-scans are recorded from a small volume of tissue or phantom, then the data is analysed subsequently, using the computer.

A-scans can also be collected from a static B-scanner which was designed to be wideband and has minimal signal processing. The RF signal from the single disc transducer is amplified and input to the transient recorder, no tgc is applied.

22.4 Experimental procedure

Attenuation estimates were made using a Diagnostic Sonar tissue-mimicking phantom. One estimate consisted of recording 40 A-scans, equispaced over a small area (1 cm by 2 cm) of the phantom. The signal was time gated so that the line began at a depth of 4 cm into the phantom. The signal was sampled at a rate of 50 MHz. The two segments of each A-line were represented by 1024 samples, corresponding to approximately 3 cm of tissue. This volume of data was thought to be equivalent to that which could be expected from a small fetal organ. A value of β was calculated for each set of 40 A-scans as described previously. The near segment and far segment log power spectra were averaged over the 40 lines before subtraction. In order to test the reproducibility of the system 32 separate estimates were made using the real-time scanner.

In addition, using the static scanner system, 32 estimates were made with each of three disc transducers having nominal centre frequencies of 3, 5 and 7 MHz.

The latter two were specially constructed to be wideband. All estimates with all transducers were made on the same volume of the phantom.

The bandwidth of each transducer was measured from the power spectrum of the echo from a reflector at the focal point of the transducer in a water bath.

22.5 Results

For each ·transducer 32 estimates of β (in dB MHz^{-1} cm^{-1}) were obtained. A histogram showing the distribution of β for each transducer is shown in *figure 22.3*. The mean values and standard deviations (SDs) are shown in *table 22.1*.

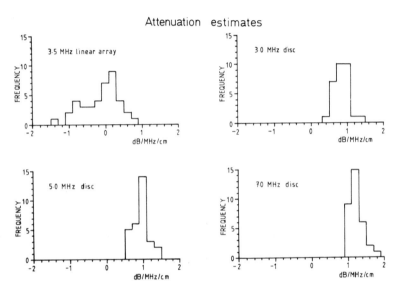

Figure 22.3 Histograms showing the distribution of β obtained with each transducer.

Table 22.1 Attenuation measurements.

Transducer	Mean β	SD
3.5 MHz linear array	−0.16	0.53
3.0 MHz disc	0.84	0.21
5.0 MHz disc	0.94	0.21
7.0 MHz disc	1.20	0.18

22.6 Discussion

The distribution of β values obtained from the real-time scanner has a large standard deviation and includes a number of negative values. Those obtained using the static scanner system have smaller SDs, and are all closer to the nominal

168

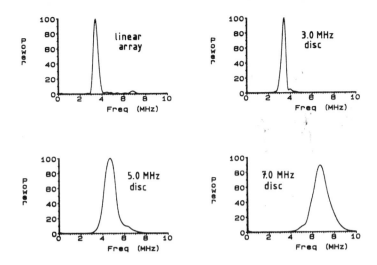

Figure 22.4 Power spectra of the transmitter pulses for each of the transducers used.

value of 1.2 dB MHz^{-1} cm^{-1} claimed by the manufacturer for the phantom. There are several factors which affect the accuracy of all the estimates, for example, the different amounts of diffraction and focussing associated with each transducer. However it is the precision or repeatability of each measurement that is being assessed here. What is it that causes variations in β when estimates are made on the same material, at the same point in the beam?

The real-time scanner has produced poorer estimates of β than the single transducer system. There are a number of factors which can affect the precision of the estimates, notably the transducer bandwidth, presence of noise in the data, and any processing of the signal that occurs between transducer and transient recorder.

The wider the bandwidth of the transducer, the more data is included in the least squares slope estimation. *Figure 22.4* shows the power spectra of the transmitted pulses for each of the four transducers used. These were obtained as described previously. The linear array and 3.0 MHz disc transducers have very narrow bandwidths, less than 1 MHz at half maximum. The 5.0 and 7.0 MHz transducers have bandwidths of nearly 2 MHz. Thus for these latter two there are nearly twice as many data points in the least squares slope estimation, and so more consistent estimates would be expected from these two.

Noise in the power spectra of the data arises from a number of sources, quantisation noise in the analogue to digital conversion, electrical noise from the scanner circuitry, and statistical noise due to averaging over too small a data set. Quantisation noise is kept to a minimum by the computer which controls the transient recorder. The computer monitors the signal level and adjusts the input range of the recorder in order to maintain as near full scale deflection as possible.

To assess the electrical noise in each scanner a measurement of signal/noise was made as follows; 40 A-scan lines were recorded at a depth of 4 cm into the phantom and the average RMS signal amplitude calculated. With all amplifier settings unchanged, 40 more A-scans were recorded with the transducer held in air so that there was no returning echo signal. There was still a detectable signal at the transient recorder due to noise in the system. The RMS signal amplitude of this electrical noise was calculated and a signal to noise ratio obtained.

The results (*table 22.2*) show that the real-time scanner produces much more electrical noise than the single transducer system, in spite of considerable efforts to improve matters. This noise arises mainly from radiation by the extensive digital

Table 22.2   Signal to noise figures.

	Real-Time Scanner	Static B Scanner
S/N	3.0	4.5

circuitry, and can be seen clearly in the power spectra obtained using that machine (*figure 22.5*). In particular the presence of the 13 MHz clock signal, which provides timing for the scanners A/D converter and CPU can be seen, along with its subharmonics. Most significantly the spikes of noise can be seen within the bandwidth of the transducer, and these will degrade the estimate of β. *Figure 22.6* shows typical spectra from the single transducer system. Although there is some low frequency noise there are not the same sharp spikes within the bandwidth of the transducer.

The real-time scanner circuitry contains an integral bandpass filter, the centre frequency of which sweeps down with depth. It was not possible to remove this from the signal path. It is difficult to assess the contribution of the scanner front-end circuitry to the overall signal characteristics, but the net effect will be to modify the intrinsic bandwidth of the transducer.

So far the discussion has considered factors which degrade the estimates of the linear array transducer relative to those of the static scanner. A further important point is that the estimates from the static scanner are not themselves sufficiently precise to consider using the system in clinical application to fetal lung. From preliminary published results[4] it would appear that an improvement of at least a factor of 2 in the standard deviation of the measured attenuation is needed in order to distinguish changes in maturing fetal lung. In spite of considerable study, the theory of backscattering from a realistic medium is not yet adequately understood. The finite transducer surface sampling an extended region of tissue is subject to interference and diffraction effects which may affect the detected signal in random or systematic ways.

We had assumed that averaging over a large number of spatial samples would reduce errors sufficiently to provide a precise estimate of the spectra of the interrogating pulse. However, these observations show that both the random effects on the distribution of spectral energy and systematic spatial variations are larger than expected. It appeared from some preliminary measurements that a significantly larger set of data may be necessary, for example using larger tissue depths. It is clear that a better understanding of the interactions involved and of methods of combining samples is needed.

We have assumed in this work that the phantom material used presents a spatially uniform attenuation. There is no means of verifying this in the present phantom. If it happens that there are small inhomogeneities, then the precision of our measurements will be better than that reported. However, it will still be the case that the linear array gives results much less precise than the disc transducer.

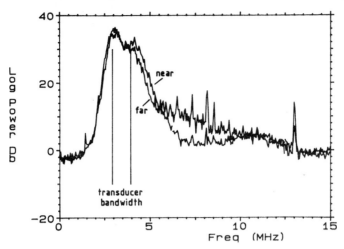

Figure 22.5 Typical log power spectra obtained using the real time scanner (averaged over 40 A-scan lines).

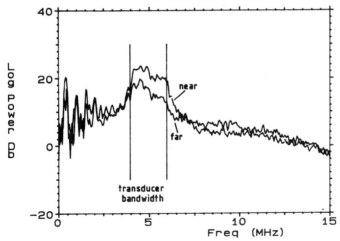

Figure 22.6 Typical log power spectra obtained using the static scanner with 5 MHz disc transducer (averaged over 40 A-scan lines).

The effects of tissue structure correlations in real organs are bound to produce systematic effects in the backscattered signal which further reduce the precision, possibly below that obtained from the phantom material.

22.7 Conclusions

The low noise, wide bandwidth requirements for attenuation measurements have not been met by the real-time linear array scanner used for these experiments. Part of the limitation is due to the particular electronic configuration which could, no doubt, be improved upon in a purpose-built instrument, and part to the intrinsically lower bandwidth of an array transducer. A disc transducer system has intrinsically better bandwidth, but a static scanner will be subject to errors of interrogating the tissue region under study, which may completely offset the improved bandwidth. Possible alternative configurations include mounting a single disc transducer on the linear array or the use of oscillating or rotating-head-transducer real time systems. However, even with the wide-band disc transducers available to our B-scanner, results are not sufficiently precise to envisage clinical use on studies of fetal lung maturity.

It is apparent that the sampling of much larger volumes of tissue is necessary for reliable use of the technique. Further work is needed to ascertain exactly how much sampling is necessary and how this may vary from organ to organ. Small organs may be unsuitable for attenuation estimates due to the limited amount of data that can be obtained from them.

Acknowledgement

The funding of this work by the Sir Jules Thorn Trust is gratefully acknowledged.

References

1 OPHIR J, SHAWKER T H, MAKLAD N F, MILLER J G, FLAX S W, NARAYANA P A and JONES J P 1984 Attenuation estimation in reflection: progress and prospects *Ultrasound Imaging* **6** 349–395
2 KUC R and SCHWARTZ M 1979 Estimating the acoustic attenuation slope for liver from reflected ultrasound signals *IEEE Trans Sonics Ultrason* **SU 26** 353–362
3 BENSON D M, WALDROP L D, KURTZ A B, ROSE J L, RIFKIN M D and GOLDBERG B B 1983 Ultrasonic tissue characterisation of fetal lung, liver and placenta for the purpose of assessing fetal maturity *J Ultrasound Med* **2** 489–494
4 MEYER C R, HERRON D S, CARSON P L, BANJAVIC R A, THIEME G A, BOOKSTEIN F L and JOHNSON M L 1984 Estimation of ultrasonic attenuation and mean backscatterer size via digital signal processing *Ultrasonic Imaging* **6** 13–23
5 LELE P P, MANSFIELD A B, MURPHY A I, NAMERY J and SENAPATI N 1975 Tissue characterisation by ultrasonic frequency-dependent attenuation and scattering *Ultrasonic Tissue Characterisation* NBS Special Publication 453 167–196
6 KUC R 1984 Estimating acoustic attenuation from reflected ultrasound signals: comparison of Spectral-shift and Spectral-difference approaches *IEEE Trans Acoustics Speech Sig Proc* **ASSP 32** 1–6

CHAPTER 23

Automatic Swept Gain in Ultrasonic Imaging

S D Pye, W N McDicken, S R Wild and T Anderson
*Departments of Medical Physics and Medical Engineering and Radiology,
Western General Hospital, Edinburgh EH4 2XU*

23.1 Introduction

The swept gain controls of most ultrasound scanners have two main limitations: they are designed to correct for attenuation in homogeneous tissue and they require time to set up correctly. In real-time scanning where the plane of scan is altered quickly, and with the use of higher frequency probes, inaccuracy in the swept gain settings has increased. The errors involved are not small — for example with 5 MHz ultrasound the attenuation compensation for a 1 cm layer of liquid should be around 10 dB less than for a 1 cm layer of soft tissue.

23.2 Clinical trials

Since ultrasonic equipment can measure the average rate of decrease of echo size with depth, it is possible to set up the gain compensation automatically[1,2]. Automatic swept gain has been somewaht neglected, probably due to a lack of clinical confirmation of its value and reliability. The authors have undertaken two clinical evaluation trials, one in obstetrics[3] and the other in the upper abdomen[4]. The automatic swept gain system used was a commercial unit manufactured by G.L. Ultrasound Ltd. which operates by measuring the average signal level within each of twelve different depth ranges. The gain settings are then adjusted so that the average signal level from each of the depth ranges is approximately the same, given the restriction that the gain must change smoothly with depth. Thus this system assumes that the tissues scanned have uniform backscattering and reflectivity rather than uniform attenuation. The trial in obstetrics showed that the image quality was improved in 45 per cent of cases and equalled that of the manual gain in another 45 per cent. Slight degradatio, due to noise, was encountered in 10 per cent of the images where large amounts of fluid were present in the uterus. In addition, the number of control manipulations was reduced by a factor of four. The results for the upper abdomen were similar to those encountered in obstetrics. Again, 90 per cent of the automatic images were at least as good as those of the manual gain. Subtle image features such as image contract changes due to metastases in the liver were not lost with the automatic system. The differences between the automatic and manual swept gain images were less marked in this trial since there were fewer collections of fluid in the scan planes.

23.3 Digital swept gain system

Developments in digital electronics now allow powerful methods of gain control to be implemented. A microcomputer controlled system has been constructed with which it is possible to store echo data and set up the swept gain automatically. The micro system is linked to a real-time mechanical sector scanner via an interface in which echo and swept gain data can be stored digitally. This system permits more localised gain compensation than present commercial systems since it allows a unique swept gain function to be generated for each line in the image. A block diagram of the system is shown in *figure 23.1*.

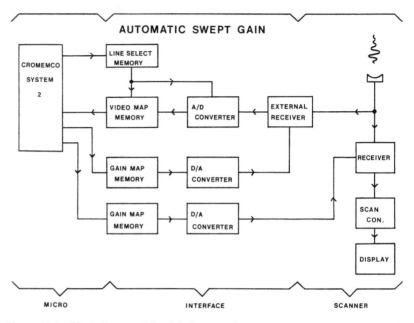

Figure 23.1   Block diagram of the digital swept gain system.

23.4   Collecting the echo data

The micro system can read from an I/O port the number of ultrasound lines in the image. It then selects up to 32 lines from which echo data will be digitised. The data is stored in a block of memory (the video map) in the interface between the microcomputer and the scanner. The signal to be digitised is taken from the input of the RF receiver inside the scanner and amplified by a second receiver in the interface. The video signal from the output of this receiver is then digitised to eight bits at 4 MHz. This corresponds to sampling the echo signal at 0.2 mm intervals down to a depth of 200 mm.

23.5   Processing the echo data

The stored echo data is processed by a Z80 microcomputer using assembly language and Fortran IV. The swept gain functions generated are stored in two blocks of memory (the gain maps) in the interface. One gain map controls the gain of the receiver in the scanner, the other controls the gain of the receiver in the interface. Each gain map can hold information for a maximum of 256 ultrasound lines. The swept gain function for each line consists of 64 eight bit values, and each value is applied for an interval corresponding to 3 mm down to a depth of 200 mm.

23.6 Speed of operation

During real-time scanning, the field of view is constantly changing. Any gain control system should be able to respond to these changes. Several features were included in the design of the digital system to improve its response time:

(i) The video map and gain map memories are part of the microcomputer memory and can be read and written to directly.

(ii) After the scan lines to be digitised have been selected by the micro the data collection is carried out by the interface independently of the micro, which can continue with other tasks.

(iii) Data in the gain maps has to be read out regularly to the receivers. The micro also needs to access the gain maps to update them. In order to avoid a conflict, and unnecessary delay to the micro, a one line buffer memory is used between each gain map and its receiver. Before being output to the receiver, each line of data is read at 4 MHz into the buffer. After a transmission pulse the data is read out of the buffer at 250 kHz, via a D/A converter, to the receiver. The maximum delay to the micro is thus only the 16 μs needed to load the buffer.

23.7 Conclusions

The clinical trials carried out so far indicate that automatic gain control can have considerable benefits: improved diagnostic images; less time spent adjusting controls; and fewer problems in staff training. The digital gain control system is now operational and will be used to study methods of deriving swept gain functions and the effect of swept gain on resolution and with different frequencies of ultrasound. The system will be tested clinically in abdominal and obstetric scanning.

References

1 McDICKEN W N, EVANS D H and ROBERTSON D A R 1974 Automatic sensitivity control in diagnostic ultrasonics *Ultrasonics* 12 173–176
2 DE CLERCQ A and MAGINNESS M G 1975 Adaptive gain control for dynamic ultrasound imaging *IEEE Ultrasonics Symposium Proceedings* 1975 IEEE Cat No 75 CHO 994–4SU (New York) 59–63
3 PYE S D, WILD S R, McDICKEN W N, ASHFORD S, ELLIOTT V, MacNAMARA A and MILLAR D 1983 A clinical trial of automatic gain control in obstetric ultrasonics *British Journal of Radiology* 56 964–968
4 PYE S D, WILD S R, McDICKEN W N and MONTGOMERY H 1985 A clinical trial of automatic gain control in abdominal ultrasound *British Journal of Radiology* 58 869–871

The Lithotripter—a Non-Invasive Method for the Disintegration of Renal Stones by Extracorporeally Generated Shock Waves

A J Coleman and J E Saunders

Medical Physics Department, St Thomas' Hospital, London SE1 7EH

24.1 Introduction

The treatment of kidney stones using extracorporeal shock wave lithotripsy (ESWL) is now performed in around 50 urology centres worldwide using the Dornier Lithotripter[1,2]. This machine was developed in the Federal Republic of West Germany by the Dornier company and the first patient was treated there in 1980. At present this is the only commercial ESWL machine in clinical operation. The results presented here have been obtained during the first three months operation of the Dornier Lithotripter at St Thomas' Hospital.

24.2 Treatment

An underwater electrical discharge is generated across an electrode gap which is positioned at the focus (F1) of a hemi-ellipsoidal reflector (semi-major axis $a = 13.8$ cm, semi-minor axis $b = 7.75$ cm) and the resulting shock wave is focused external to the ellipsoid at F2. The patient is suspended on a moveable support in a bath of de-gassed, softened water and a stereoscopic X-ray fluoroscopy system is used to position the patient so that the kidney stone is located at the focus (F2) where sufficient pressure is developed to disintegrate the stone. A complete treatment consists of around 1500 shocks which are triggered by the R-wave of the ECG. The electrodes require replacement after 700 shocks by which time the initial electrode gap of 0.4 mm has increased to about 2 mm due to erosion.

24.3 Measurements

A high pressure, quartz crystal transducer with a diameter of 6 mm has been used to measure the pressure around the focus (F2). The variations in peak pulse pressure produced by the focused shock wave along the major axis of the ellipsoid through F2 and parallel to the minor axis through F2 are plotted in *figure 24.1* and *figure 24.2* respectively for a discharge potential DP equal to 20 kV. The relative peak pressure is given by the peak voltage produced by the transducer as measured on an oscilloscope. The transducer output corresponds to a peak pressure (P_m) of approximately 33 MPa at F2 which is found to vary linearly with discharge potential over the range 15 kV to 25 kV where $P_m = 4.59 + 1.42DP$ (DP in kV, P_m in MPa). These absolute pressure values should be regarded with caution as they are based on a static calibration whereas the transducer in the present situation is measuring a transient pressure. The full width half maxima (FWHM)

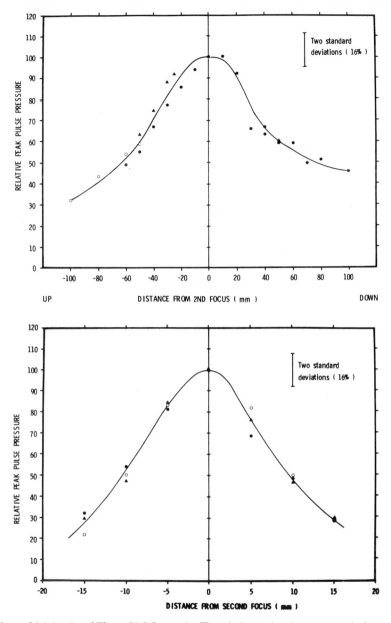

Figure 24.1 (top) and **Figure 24.2** (bottom)   The relative peak pulse pressure of a focused shock wave generated underwater, measured using a quartz crystal transducer (6 mm diameter) at positions along the major axis (top) and minor axis (bottom) through the focus (F2) of an ellipsoidal reflector. Each point is the mean of ten readings. The three types of symbol used for data points represent readings taken on different occasions using different electrodes.

of the peak pressure distribution in the major and minor axis directions are 12 cm and 2 cm respectively. These values are larger than those previously published by Chaussy[1] who gives a FWHM(major axis)=1.7 cm and FWHM(minor axis)=0.6 cm for an ellipsoid with a=11 cm and b=7.8 cm. The shock waves produce an effect on the surface of the water which may be visually observed. Within 7 cm either side of the geometrical location of F2 along the major axis, this effect raises a narrow column of water above the surface. This tends to confirm our findings on the width of the pressure distribution. P_m was observed to rise slowly as the electrode gap increased with age up to about 1000 shocks and decrease rapidly thereafter due to the difficulty in obtaining a proper discharge. The pressure-time curve measured at F2 showed a small peak in advance of the main focused wave which was produced by the direct (unfocused) shock wave. The main (focused) wave rose steeply to a peak pressure which was about twenty-five times that of the direct wave. The FWHM of the pressure pulse with respect to time as measured by the transducer increased from approximately 1.4 to 1.8 μs as the DP was raised from 15 to 24 kV. These figures should be used with caution in view of the rise time (10 per cent–90 per cent) of the transducer being of the same order as these times i.e. 1 μs.

24.4 Noise

There is a loud crack associated with each electrical discharge which is a potential hazard for personnel working with the equipment. Measurements at the St Thomas' site indicate RMS sound pressure levels during the shock wave pulse of about 90 dB at 2 m from the bath and 93 dB at the patient's head[3]. When corrected for the response of the human ear, the typical level to which staff will be exposed is estimated to be 84 dB(A). These values are about 4 dB higher without a patient in the bath. With a repetition frequency of about one per second, the 150 ms duration airborne sound pulse is not considered to be as damaging as a continuous sound of the same amplitude, but information about effects of pulsed sound is limited and it could be misleading simply to average the pressure over the total treatment time or even the working day. Staff and patients are advised to wear ear protection and the treatment room is specially sound insulated to limit disturbance to nearby rooms.

24.5 Radiation dose

The radiation dose to the patient from the X-ray localisation procedure has been measured for 33 patients using LiF TLD dosimeters placed on the skin at the entry point at each of the two beams. The mean skin dose of the 33 patients was found to be 12 cGy with a range of 2 cGy–53 cGy, comparable to doses received from screening in cardiac catheterisation procedures.

24.6 Biological effects

Biological effects are known to occur with high power ultrasound and are to be expected in ESWL. Erythema is noted on the skin of many patients at the entry and exit points of the shock wave. Haematuria and renal colic are relatively frequent side effects of the treatment. The treatment is known to be painful and all patients are anaesthetised, 50 per cent using an epidural catheter and 50 per cent by general anaesthetic.

References

1 CHAUSSY C (Ed) 1982 *Extra corporeal shock wave lithotripsy* (Karger, Basle)
2 WICKHAM J E A *et al* 1985 Extra corporeal shock wave lithotripsy: the first 50 patients treated in Britain *Br med J* **290** 1188–1189
3 FROST G P 1985 *Summary of noise measurements on the Lithotripter installation at St Thomas' Hospital* Personal communication

CONTRIBUTORS

Dr D R Bacon

Senior Scientific Officer
Division of Radiation Science and Acoustics
National Physics Laboratory
Teddington, Middlesex TW11 0LW

Dr D C Barber

Principal Physicist
Department of Medical Physics and Clinical
   Engineering
Royal Hallamshire Hospital
Glossop Road
Sheffield S10 2JF

Dr A J Coleman

Senior Physicist
Physics Department
St. Thomas's Hospital
Lambeth Palace Road
London SE1 7EH

Mr G Cusick

Principal Physicist
Department of Medical Physics and
   Bioengineering
University College Hospital
1st Fl–Shropshire House
11–20 Capper Street
London WC1E 6JA

Dr L E Drain

Principal Scientific Officer
Atomic Energy Research Establishment
Harwell
Oxfordshire OX11 0RA

Dr F A Duck

Top Grade Physicist
Medical Physics Department
Royal United Hospital
Combe Park
Bath BA1 3NG

Dr M Dyson

Senior Lecturer
Department of Anatomy
Guy's Hospital
London SE1 9RT

Dr D H Evans

Principal Physicist
Department of Medical Physics and Clinical
   Engineering
Leicester Royal Infirmary
Leicester LE1 5WW

180

Dr J A Evans	Lecturer Department of Medical Physics University of Leeds Leeds General Infirmary Leeds LS1 3EX
Dr J M Evans	Senior Physicist Medical Physics Department Bristol General Hospital 1–2 Redcliffe Parade West Bristol BS1 6SP
Mr D H Follett	Principal Physicist Medical Physics Department Electronics Development Unit Bristol General Hospital 1–2 Redcliffe Parade West Bristol BS1 6SP
Mr J E Gardener	Department of Medical Physics and Bio-engineering University College Hospital 11–20 Capper Street London WC1E 6JA
Mr A J Hawkins	Physics Student Medical Physics Department Royal United Hospital Bath BA1 3NG
Dr S Leeman	Senior Lecturer Department of Medical Engineering and Physics King's College School of Medicine and Dentistry Denmark Hill London SE5
Mr D J Locke	Physicist Bioengineering Unit University Hospital of Wales Heath Park Cardiff CF4 4XW
Dr M J Lunt	Top Grade Physicist Poole General Hospital Longfleet Road Poole Dorset BH15 2JB

Mr K McCarty	Principal Physicist Bioengineering Unit University Hospital of Wales Heath Park Cardiff CF4 4XW
Dr W N McDicken	Top Grade Physicist Department of Medical Physics and Medical Engineering Royal Infirmary Edinburgh EH3 9YW
Mr D J McHugh	Principal Physicist Regional Department of Medical Physics Christie Hospital Wilmslow Road Manchester M20 9BX
Mr R J Marsh	Physicist Department of Medical Physics and Bio-Engineering University College Hospital 1st Fl–Shropshire House 11–20 Capper Street London WC1E 6JA
Dr K Martin	Senior Physicist Regional Medical Physics Department Newcastle General Hospital Westgate Road Newcastle-upon-Tyne NE4 6BE
Dr B C Moss	Senior Scientific Officer Atomic Energy Research Establishment Harwell Oxfordshire OX11 0RA
Mr D Peake	Medical Physics Technician Medical Physics Department Electronics Development Unit Bristol General Hospital 1–2 Redcliffe Parade West Bristol BS1 6SP
Dr J M Pelmore	Senior Physicist Medical Physics Department Leicester Royal Infirmary Infirmary Square Leicester LE1 5WW

Dr R C Preston	Principal Scientific Officer National Physical Laboratory Teddington Middlesex TW11 0LW
Mr R Price	Principal Physicist Medical Physics Department The General Infirmary Leeds LS1 3EX
Mr W I J Pryce	Principal Physicist Department of Medical Physics and Clinical Engineering Northern General Hospital Herries Road Sheffield S5 7AU
Dr S Pye	Department of Medical Physics and Medical Engineering and Radiology Western General Hospital Edinburgh EH4 2XU
Miss R E Richardson	Principal Physicist Medical Physics Department City Hospital Hucknall Road Nottingham NG5 1PB
Mr T J Roberts	Physicist Regional Medical Physics Department Newcastle General Hospital Westgate Road Newcastle-upon-Tyne NE4 6BE
Professor V C Roberts	Professor of Medical Electronics Department of Medical Engineering and Physics King's College School of Medicine and Dentistry Denmark Hill London SE5
Mr T E Saunders	Principal Physicist Medical Physics Department St. Thomas's Hospital Lambeth Palace Road London SE1 7EH
Miss S B Sherriff	Senior Physicist Department of Medical Physics and Clinical Engineering Royal Hallamshire Hospital Glossop Road Sheffield S10 2JF

Dr R Skidmore	Top Grade Physicist Medical Physics Department Bristol General Hospital Guinea Street Bristol BS1 6SY
Dr R A Smith	Scientific Officer National Physics Laboratory Teddington Middlesex TW11 0LW
Miss H C Starritt	Senior Physicist Medical Physics Department Royal United Hospital Combe Park Bath SA1 3NG
Dr W F Tait	Surgical Registrar University Department of Surgery Withington Hospital Manchester M20
Professor P N T Wells	Professor of Radiodiagnosis Medical Physics Department Bristol General Hospital Guinea Street Bristol BS1 6SY
Dr T A Whittingham	Top Grade Physicist Regional Medical Physics Department Newcastle General Hospital Newcastle-upon-Tyne NE4 6BE
Dr S R Wild	Consultant Radiologist Department of Medical Physics and Medical Engineering and Radiology Western General Hospital Edinburgh EH4 2XU
Dr K Wilson	Principal Physicist Bio-engineering Department St. Thomas's Hospital Lambeth Palace Road London SE1 7EH
Dr B Zeqiri	Higher Scientific Officer National Physical Laboratory Teddington Middlesex TW11 0LW